Genetic politics
From eugenics to genome

Anne Kerr and Tom Shakespeare
with cartoons by Suzy Varty

D0879551

New Clarion Press

Issues in Social Policy

Dedicated to Rosa, James, Ivy and Robert with love

First published 2002

New Clarion Press
5 Church Row, Gretton
Cheltenham GL54 5HG
England

New Clarion Press is a workers' co-operative.

A catalogue record for this book is available from the British Library.

ISBN   paperback   1 873797 25 7
           hardback   1 873797 26 5

Typeset in 10/12 Times New Roman by Jean Wilson Typesetting, Coventry

Printed in Great Britain by MFP Design and Print, Manchester

Contents

Acknowledgements

We would like to thank Chris Bessant at New Clarion Press for his patience and faith in our abilities to finally complete this project. Many thanks also to Sarah Cunningham-Burley, Nick Watson, Bill Albert, Agnes Fletcher and all the folk at PEALS for ongoing discussions about genetics, disability and society. Brian Woods deserves a special mention for his love and support. Michael Whong-Barr read and commented on earlier drafts of the manuscript, and we gratefully acknowledge his help. Thanks also to Suzy Varty for the cartoons. We would also like to acknowledge the work of many scholars on which we draw here, in particular Adrienne Asch, Michael Burleigh, Angus Clarke, Ruth Hubbard, Daniel Kevles, Rayna Rapp, Barbara Katz Rothman, Dorothy Nelkin, Abby Lippman, Diane Paul and Hilary and Steven Rose. If this book has but a fraction of the impact of their work on our understanding of eugenics, genetics and society, it will be a success. Anne would also like to acknowledge the financial support provided by the Wellcome Trust History of Medicine Programme during the period of writing.

Anne Kerr and Tom Shakespeare

The cover photograph shows a demonstration organized by eugenic campaigners outside the office of the editor of the *Medical Review of Reviews* on Wall Street, New York, 1915. Reproduced by kind permission of the State Historical Society of Wisconsin, negative no. WHi (X3) 14579.

Abbreviations

ABI	Association of British Insurers
ACGT	Advisory Commission on Gene Testing
ASHG	American Society for Human Genetics
CMGS	Clinical Molecular Genetics Society
DNA	deoxyribonucleic acid
ELSI	Ethical, Legal and Social Implications Programme
EU	European Union
FDA	Food and Drug Administration
GAIC	Genetics and Insurance Committee
HFEA	Human Fertilization and Embryology Authority
HFEB	Human Fertilization and Embryology Bill
HGC	Human Genetics Commission
HGP	Human Genome Project
HUGO	Human Genome Organization
IVF	in vitro fertilization
NHS	National Health Service
NIH	National Institutes of Health
'OGOD'	one gene, one disease
PGD	pre-implantation genetic diagnosis
PKU	phenylketonuria
RAC	Recombinant DNA Molecule Professional Advisory Committee
rDNA	recombinant DNA
SNP	single nucleotide polymorphism
USPTO	United States Patent and Trademark Office

1
Introduction

We are poised at a turning point of human history. Behind us lies a twentieth century marked by unprecedented technological developments, but also the nightmares of human barbarism and war. In front of us stretches 'the century of the gene', when we are promised that science will be harnessed for the common good: to reduce the impact of disease, to increase longevity and to provide solutions for social problems including famine and global poverty. It is a good moment to explore, in the field of genetics, what went wrong in so many countries during the first part of the twentieth century, and to ask whether we are currently repeating some of the mistakes of the past, or growing problems for the future.

This book provides a general introduction to the social context of human genetics. In the first six chapters, we review the history of attempts to control human reproduction via policies of eugenics during the twentieth century. In Chapters 7–11, we explore the growth and implications of human genomics. Genomics involves sequencing and characterizing the genome, commonly referred to as our genetic code. The identification of genes associated with disease is of paramount importance, through diagnostic tests and larger screening programmes, but so is the development of genetic and pharmaceutical treatments for genetic diseases. We consider these developments as well as their social consequences and the cultural understandings and representations of genetics, disability and disease that they involve. The first part of the book largely summarizes existing secondary literature for the benefit of newcomers to the field; the second part develops our own analysis of the contemporary situation.

'Genetic politics' covers a vast field that is rapidly changing. This has meant we have had to be selective. From the start, we have excluded consideration of non-human genetics, and the fields of agriculture and biotechnology. Neither have we discussed non-genetic dilemmas in bioethics, such as the contemporary debate over euthanasia. The focus is primarily on the UK, although we discuss the USA and other European countries at various points. We are particularly concerned by the

1

implications of genetic developments for disabled people, and are less focused on the implications of genetics for ethnic minorities and indigenous
peoples, although we try to take account of some of the most pressing concerns facing these communities. Our focus on disability and genetics has
also meant that our interest extends beyond genetics in the strict sense of
the word, to screening for other chromosomal and developmental abnormalities in pregnancy. Throughout we try to direct the reader to other
sources for more in-depth analysis, particularly in the first part of the book
on the history of eugenics.

What we write in the pages that follow is inevitably marked by our own
biographies and our own political outlooks. Anne is a science graduate,
who has moved into the sociology of science and technology and has particular interests in the social and historical dimensions of genetics and
feminist analysis of science. Tom is a social scientist, whose previous
work has mainly been in the field of disability studies. He has moved into
bioethics and the public understanding of science in recent years. We are
both parents, and Tom and his family are affected by achondroplasia, a genetic form of restricted growth.

Our approaches to medical science in general, and genetics in particular,
are based on a commitment to radical critique of the cultural values and
social relationships that shape knowledge and technology. Neither of us is
'anti-science', nor do we claim that there are no such things as genes or diseases. But we take the view that knowledge and technology are not neutral.
The study of genetic diseases and the tests and treatments that are developed
to control them reflect a range of values about illness, disability and deviance, which need to be questioned rather than ignored. These practices also
involve many powerful interest groups, from senior scientists and doctors,
to the state and commercial companies. Their involvement in determining
what genetic technologies get developed and how they are regulated also
requires careful exploration and critique. In the area of reproduction, we
support a woman's right to choose, but we also support a disability rights
perspective: most impairments do not make life not worth living, and genetics is not the main solution to the problem of disability. We are
particularly concerned about the potential for discrimination on the basis
of genetic information and we believe that genetic research and applications need to be developed in the interests of people, not profit. We are also
keen to see better mechanisms for public consultation and involvement in
policy and ethical debate about genetics.

Before we go on to explore these issues in the rest of the book, we want
to say a few words about eugenics. It is a complicated concept. As Diane
Paul writes, 'Eugenics is a word with nasty connotations but an indetermi-
nate meaning.'[1] There is little disagreement about the use of the term to

describe the ideas of population improvement that were circulating in the first half of the twentieth century, or to describe the practices of sterilization and euthanasia in countries such as the USA, Germany and the Scandinavian states. However, there is less clarity as to what the word 'eugenics' strictly means, especially its applicability in the modern era. This is partly because of the widespread rhetorical deployment of the 'eugenics' label.

Those commentators and critics who are in opposition to contemporary human genetics policy and practice sometimes use the term 'eugenics' to condemn it. In this way, they draw upon a generalized revulsion towards the abuses of the pre-war period, and the extremes of Nazi euthanasia policies in particular. Sometimes critics have gone further, and have labelled geneticists as fascists or Nazis. Radicals in the disability movement have resorted to slogans such as 'No Nazi eugenics', and have called genetics 'an extermination policy' or 'a search and destroy mission directed against disabled people'.[2] The difference, for many critics, is that modern genetics is more sophisticated and can pursue policies of population improvement or racial hygiene more effectively. Arthur Caplan writes: 'One shudders to think what the use of genetic information based upon the genome might have meant in terms of social policy in Alabama in 1890, Germany in 1939, or South Africa in 1970.'[3] Although Caplan sees few problems with contemporary practices, many critics would argue that there is a continuum between the injustices he cites and the new powers of genetic intervention at the turn of the twenty-first century.

The quote from Caplan highlights the way that professionals in the genetics field and their allies have used the term 'eugenics' in order to identify 'bad science' or 'human rights abuses' and to distance themselves and their work from the abuses of the past, or from inhumane policies in non-western countries such as China. They distinguish contemporary western practice by its commitment to offering individuals and families informed choice, and by its focus on disease as opposed to social or racial groups considered to be deviant.

Yet, as will become clear in this book, we are sceptical about this rhetorical ploy. It is not possible to clearly demarcate disease from social deviance, as diseases are defined according to social attitudes about acceptable behaviour and physical and mental aptitudes. Social deviance also tends to be medicalized. It is also difficult to clearly distinguish the priorities of eugenics policies in the past from some of the priorities of contemporary genetic screening policies, where emphasis is often placed upon reducing the number of people born with genetic diseases. Angus Clarke has pointed out that many policy documents ritually disown eugenics, before going on to propose interventions that seem dangerously close to the eugenic values of the past.[4] Jo Lenaghan suggests: 'A commitment towards a human rights approach may be used to (cosmetically) distance the speaker from nasty "eugenic" abuses of genetics without altering the ethos of the service on offer.'[5] An example of this is provided by the 1991 Royal College of Physicians Report, *Purchasers' Guidelines on Genetic Services in the NHS*. Many such documents skirt around the ethos or purpose of contemporary genetic and obstetric intervention, or mask other intentions behind the veil of informed consent.

Sometimes the mask slips, when an individual makes a comment that suggests other motivations for some of these developments. For example, the pioneer of reproductive technology, Professor Bob Edwards, incautiously announced at the 1999 annual meeting of the European Society of Human Reproduction and Embryology: 'Soon it will be a sin of parents to have a child that carries the heavy burden of genetic disease. We are entering a world where we have to consider the quality of our children.'[6] While few doctors or researchers are as blatant as this in public, there are many anecdotal examples of professionals' eugenic attitudes reported by parents making reproductive choices. Other research, such as the study conducted by Anne and her colleagues at the University of Edinburgh, has shown that scientists and doctors often hold implicit eugenic values: for example, when they argue that disabled lives are not worth living, or that it is socially responsible to prevent the birth of genetically defective babies.[7] Moreover, the literature on screening often evaluates new techniques in terms of cost–benefit arguments: for example, comparing the cost of a Down's syndrome screening programme per Down's pregnancy terminated with the cost of the lifetime care of someone with Down's syndrome.[8]

Eugenics cannot be boxed off as a relic of the past. Nor can it be equated in any simple sense with the genetic medicine of the present. But is it possible to come up with a more subtle definition? The word itself was coined in 1883 by Francis Galton, a cousin of Charles Darwin, to mean 'well born'. Galton defined it as 'the science of improvement of the human germ plasm through better breeding'. It could therefore be defined broadly as 'genetic improvement'. But this might include a whole range of maternity and paediatric services, possibly the whole of genetic medicine. This stretches the definition of eugenics too far and waters down our concerns about coercion and elimination of the so-called genetically defective. Therefore it seems necessary to limit the word to attempts to intervene in the area of inheritance.

The philosopher Jonathan Glover highlights two key definitional parameters on which there seems to be consensus. First, 'If we want to keep the word for the really controversial cases, we can stipulate that a policy is

eugenic only if it has the aim of influencing the composition of the population.'[9] Second, Glover expresses a common view in another of his
publications, when he specifies further that it is not 'genetic improvement'
which is the problem, but the means by which this is achieved:

> Few people object to the uses of eugenic policies to eliminate disorders,
> unless those policies have additional features which are objectionable.
> Most of us are resistant to the use of compulsion, and those who oppose
> abortion will object to screening programmes. But apart from those
> other moral objections, we do not object to the use of eugenic policies
> against disease.[10]

This is the perspective taken by Daniel Kevles in *In the Name of Eugenics*,
when he argues that the contemporary revolution in genetics is not likely
to be used for eugenics because of our emphasis on reproductive freedom
and civil rights for disabled people, in contrast to the state-sponsored coercion of the past.

If we wish to retain a pejorative notion of eugenics, this suggests we
could reach a core definition of eugenics as the combination of a population policy to improve the genetic health of the next generation, involving
some measure of compulsion. The inhuman dimensions of such an approach lie in the suggestion that individual desires must be sacrificed to a
larger public good.

However, problems remain with this approach. First, as we will demonstrate in the first part of the book, the historical practice of eugenics
included voluntary measures to improve 'racial hygiene' as well as coercion. They also included 'positive eugenics' – extra breeding by the
'genetically healthy' – as well as 'negative eugenics' – less breeding by
the 'genetically unfit'. Diane Paul cites the British Eugenics Education
Society, which adopted the tactics of 'education, persuasion and induce-
ment' rather than law or coercion as in the American model of eugenics.[11]

Second, this approach focuses on whether a policy is designed to implement change at a population level: it assumes an agent with a goal. Most
modern genetic services are not designed with this explicit intention: they
are designed to offer couples choice in reproduction. Yet the outcome of
such an ostensibly non-eugenic approach may be a change in the composition of the population. This is what Troy Duster has called 'back door
eugenics'.[12] The philosopher Philip Kitcher intends to give a more positive
spin to the current western approach of voluntary screening programmes
plus reproductive choice by referring to it as 'consumer eugenics'.[13]
Arthur Caplan goes further, to advocate a eugenics that involves enabling
individuals voluntarily to enhance the capabilities of their offspring, not
just to restore function or correct disability, but actually to improve on

their ordinary human capacities. These values have much in common with the eugenics of the past.

Third, as we shall discuss in Chapter 8, there are powerful social and cultural forces that undermine people's autonomy, and which prevent individuals and families from exercising informed choice in the antenatal scenario. Recent research has revealed that the notion of non-directive counselling is a myth. And while the notion of patient autonomy is the dominant value of contemporary bioethics and medicine, we believe it is often illusory, given the social and cultural contexts in which all individuals find themselves located, and the pressures that influence the actions of people who are disempowered or impoverished in modern societies. This blurs the boundary between coercion in the eugenics of the past and so-called free choice in the genetics of the present.

For these reasons, we believe that eugenics is best thought of as a loose concept where the elimination of hereditary genetic disease, primarily through reproductive interventions, is emphasized, but the means by which this can be achieved are various. The most overt and problematic forms of eugenics involve large-scale population screening, coercion and controversial categories of 'disease' or disorder. But eugenics can also come in the guise of individual choice. And it can include 'genetic enhancement' as well as the elimination of disease.

A minority of obstetricians and geneticists hold explicit eugenic views about the benefits to society of preventing disabled people from being born. But rather than concentrating on these individuals, we believe it is important to examine and to challenge the system of genetics as a whole, and the social relations and cultural values which mean that genetic screening becomes a solution to the problem of disability. We therefore argue that eugenics is an 'emergent property' of the prevailing structure of reproduction. Here, the analogy is with consciousness and the brain. It is impossible to say where consciousness emerges from the brain. There is no one origin or cause of consciousness. But undoubtedly, the combination of elements in the vastly complex human brain produces consciousness as an outcome.[14] We therefore argue that the policies, practices, professionals and social contexts in which clinical genetics occurs can create an outcome that is eugenic. We disagree with Jonathan Glover and argue that there are serious moral and social problems with the drive to eliminate disease and difference at all costs. We do not believe that the world would be a better place without disabled people. Nor do we believe that disability is a tragedy best avoided. We also disagree with Arthur Caplan, and oppose the non-therapeutic use of genetics to enhance the capabilities of individuals beyond their ordinary endowment.

However, our concerns about contemporary genomics go beyond reproduction. Genetic diseases are unlikely to be eliminated through reproductive intervention. This means that contemporary genomics is also focused upon better and more frequent techniques of surveillance to be used by people with genetic disorders. Although their promise has yet to be realized, the development of genetic medicines and treatments is also a possibility. Why should we be concerned about this? Because the commercial context in which genetic research and services are being developed raises many concerns about inequality of provision, particularly the creation of a 'genetic underclass' unable to afford genetic medicines. New modes of surveillance might also be used to exercise an inappropriate level of control over people's lifestyles and behaviours. Again, just because people perform this surveillance upon themselves, it does not mean that it cannot infringe upon their freedom.

In the concluding chapter, we will outline an alternative ethos for genetics and society, concentrating on ways to undermine the potential for a new eugenics. In the intervening pages, we will document the historical experience of eugenics, and explore the contemporary approach of clinical genetics and the social contexts within which it operates. We begin with the birth of eugenics, in the UK and the USA, before moving on to consider Nazi and Scandinavian eugenics. We then turn to what Kevles has aptly called reform eugenics, tracing the reconfiguration of genetic medicine in the post-war era, to the emergence of modern genomics towards the end of the twentieth century. In the latter part of the book, we consider the implications of these developments in terms of culture, genetic choices and their wider social consequences, and the governance of genomics.

2

The rise of eugenics in the UK and the USA

The control of human heredity has a long history. The idea of 'like begets like' and the stigma and fear of disability are literally ancient. As Rosen and colleagues note in *The History of Mental Retardation*, the practices of infanticide and euthanasia of disabled children are known to have occurred since ancient Roman times. It was not until the rise of a new humanitarian spirit in the nineteenth century that state hospitals and schools were established for the 'retarded'. But the goals of these institutions gradually shifted from protection of the so-called deviants from society to protection of society from the deviants. This was the beginning of eugenics, classified by Francis Galton into two types: 'positive' eugenics, which focused on encouraging so-called good stock to breed, and 'negative' eugenics, which focused on discouraging the mentally and morally unfit from breeding.

Eugenics drew admirers from a wide swathe of the professional middle classes at the turn of the century. The scientific and medical professions were its mainstay. Geneticists deserve a special mention, as their emergent discipline was not only motivated in many ways by eugenic concerns, it also gave scientific weight to eugenics in the form of theory and 'evidence'. Although this became increasingly dubious by the standards of the time, some important genetic techniques and theories owe their origin to eugenics: thus genetics and eugenics cannot be easily disentangled. Indeed, the story of early eugenics is one of the best ways of illustrating the profoundly social aspects of science and technology that are all too often ignored.

This chapter will start by exploring the social and political background to early eugenics, before moving on to consider its links to the beginnings of the science of genetics and its relationship to the broader scientific and medical communities. We will focus on how eugenics shaped the themes and forms of science and medicine. We then broaden our focus to consider the popular movements that physicians and scientists spearheaded in the promotion of eugenics. The various strategies to popularize eugenics and its implementation in the notorious sterilization programmes of the USA and the institutionalization of the 'mentally defective' in the USA and UK are also discussed.

Social turmoil: the background to early eugenics

The turn of the century was a period of considerable social turmoil in both Britain and the USA. The growth of capitalism brought with it industrial unrest and urban slums. In Britain, concern was mounting about national efficiency and population degeneracy. The growing numbers of the urban poor and the poor physical condition of recruits for the Boer War (1899–1902) stimulated particular anxieties about deterioration of the national physique. There were also concerns about the declining birth rate amongst the middle classes and the unrestrained reproduction of the 'unfit' amongst the lower classes. In response, the middle classes expanded government and regulation and looked to impartial scientific experts to manage society.

There was also a shift towards state responsibility for welfare and a growth in charities around this time. In Britain, the Metropolitan Poor Act (1867) and the Idiots Act (1886) marked the beginnings of the wide-scale institutionalization of people considered to be socially and mentally inadequate: the so-called imbeciles, idiots, lunatics and feeble-minded. In practice, a wide range of mental and physical disabilities and conditions were actually grouped together under this heading, including microcephaly, epilepsy and 'Mongolism' (which is known as Down's syndrome today). Poor sight or hearing and even left-handedness were also used to make a diagnosis. Institutionalization was favoured because these groups were considered to be in need of special treatment, not available in the community. As Thomson has argued in *The Problem of Mental Deficiency*, mental deficiency became a social problem.

As the hereditary explanation for feeble-mindedness drew force, so too did an understanding of the hereditary basis of criminality. In the USA institutions such as asylums and prisons expanded and concerns about their costs grew, as did doubts about the prospects for curing the inmates. Humans were viewed no longer as the 'masters of their own destiny', but as prone to influence by the environment and, most particularly, their heredity.

Scientists also began to professionalize during this period, and science became institutionalized in the universities. Biologists were keen to establish themselves alongside their colleagues in the physical sciences, and adopted the 'hard' techniques of experiment and mechanistic explanations in its pursuit. Medicine too was developing a scientific approach and physicians' status was growing. A new middle class of professionals was therefore emerging.

Early genetics, science and medicine

The 'new biology' of this era also contributed to a new sense of genetic determinism. This involved microscopic studies of the cell and early statistics. August Weismann's theory of the germ plasm (which replaced the Lamarckian emphasis on the inheritance of acquired characteristics), the reinterpretation of Gregor Mendel's theories in terms of dominant and recessive genes, and Hugo De Vries' mutation theory of evolution undermined the environmental determinism of the previous years. As Kaye has argued in *The Social Meaning of Modern Biology*, a new pessimism about social change arose as the immutability of genes was emphasized.

Two branches of early genetics developed simultaneously: biometry and Mendelianism. Biometry, favoured by Francis Galton, stressed the importance of a series of small steps in inheritance. Mendelianism, favoured by William Bateson, emphasized its discontinuous character. These two branches of early genetics were both linked to eugenics in a number of ways. Biometricians and Mendelians studied the inheritance of albinism, alcoholism, insanity, tuberculosis, mental defects and criminality. Galton, and his successor Karl Pearson, set up the Eugenics Laboratory in the University of London in 1907. Here they sought to establish eugenics as a science. Their studies involved extensive research into the mental and physical characteristics of populations. Biometricians' rationale of prediction was intimately tied to their aims of social control and the planned improvement of the population. Charles Davenport, who subsequently 'defected' to Mendelianism, also established the Eugenics Record Office in the USA, and conducted extensive research into the inheritance of a vast array of characteristics and ailments. Mendelians were also motivated by eugenic concerns. For example, Donald MacKenzie notes that although Bateson found the programme of race improvement distasteful, he viewed class differences in genetic terms.[1]

Although eugenicists are often ridiculed for some of their more outlandish claims, they also made some important contributions to the study of inheritance. Galton and Pearson developed the correlation coefficient, and the 'bell curve' of normal distribution, both major tools in statistics. In

No Other Gods, Charles Rosenberg notes that Davenport and his wife, Gertrude, were the first to apply the concept of polygenic inheritance to a human trait (skin colour) and to explain eye colour in terms of multiple alternative genes.[2]

Other medical research, which has since been incorporated into the canon of genetic research, also bolstered eugenics in this period. Archibald Garrod's work on *Inborn Errors of Metabolism* (1908) gave geneticists the confidence that Mendel's laws could be applied to humans as well as plants, and spurred their interest in a broader range of more common traits. Even the ultimate resolution of biometry and Mendelianism in the population genetics of the 1930s, which is often taken to mark the break between genetics and eugenics, can be linked to eugenics. Kevles shows that despite his later efforts to distance himself from eugenics, one of the principal protagonists, R. A. Fisher, was clearly motivated by a concern to turn science to the improvement of the population, as he wrote in his essay of 1914, 'Some hopes of a eugenicist'.

The links between genetics and eugenics go beyond the motivation of key scientists, however. Geneticists' professional associations, such as the American Genetics Associations, and funding bodies, including the Rockefeller Foundation, supported eugenics. Eugenics also inspired a new generation of scientists, in the USA in particular. As Paul notes, by 1914, 44 American colleges and universities offered courses in eugenics. The number rose to 376 by 1928.[3] Many other scientists (including social scientists) were also supportive of eugenics in this era. Eugenics was intimately associated with the emerging discipline of psychology. For example, the Binet test (the forerunner to the IQ test) was introduced in the USA in 1910 at a time when psychologists were seeking professional recognition. This did much to reinforce the hereditarian view of mental capacity, especially theories of racial and class differences in intelligence. Lowe also writes that, in Britain, many psychologists, school doctors and educators of the early twentieth century embraced eugenics, chiming as it did with their preoccupations with the dangers of the urban poor. IQ tests were used to identify feeble-minded schoolchildren, who were then removed to special schools, as authorized in the Mental Deficiency Act of 1913. Members of the Board of Education were also at the forefront of calls for a Royal Commission to investigate sterilization. As Lowe documents, in 1929 the executive of the National Union of Teachers even approved a resolution which stated that 'the time is now right for a scientific enquiry into the whole question of reproduction among the mentally defective'.[4]

Notwithstanding a general disinterest in genetics amongst the medical profession, and a preference for environmental explanations for disease, Thomson notes that *The Lancet* and the Royal College of Surgeons and

Physicians both made statements in support of eugenic sterilization. Indeed, as Farrall has argued,[5] it was 'medical men' who were at the forefront of calls for negative eugenics. Thomson also argues that psychiatrists took up hereditarian theories at this time in an effort to explain their lack of success in curing the increasing numbers of the mentally ill. Medical professionals such as eye specialists and surgeons were also attracted to the eugenics movement's proposals to legalize the sterilization of people who were thought to be carriers of genetic defects. Several leading physicians in the USA also played an important role in securing the passage of sterilization legislation. Indeed, without medical professionals, the widespread practices of sterilization, which we go on to discuss below, would not have been possible.

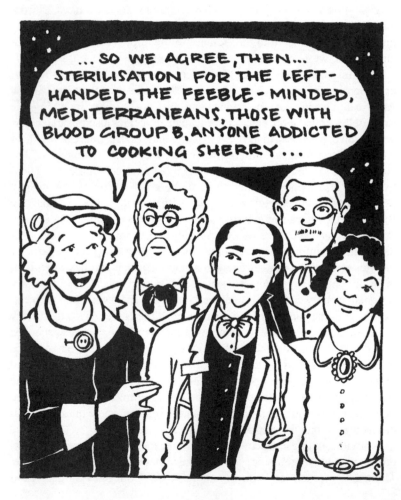

What is clear, however, is that eugenics was (and is) not a unified ideology or science. As Farrall notes of this period: 'Not even the biological community had one understanding of "evolution" or "natural selection" or "heredity"; how then could such a wide-ranging group as those who wrote on "eugenics" be expected to have identical understandings of what eugenics stood for?'[6] But, the logical inconsistencies of eugenics presented no barrier to its popular appeal.

The eugenics movements and popular support

The first organization in the eugenics movement, the Eugenics Education Society, was set up in Britain in 1907. Inspired by Galton, the membership shifted from 'gentlemanly amateurs' in its first decade to the professional middle classes in its second. Psychiatrists, physicians and academics dominated the society in this era, with women accounting for half the membership. Although the membership reached only 700 at its peak, it did include the academic elite in its membership and had wider appeal amongst this group. As Kevles notes,

> In 1911 the Oxford University Union moved approval of the principles of eugenics by a vote of almost two to one, and meetings of a eugenics society at Cambridge University before the war drew hundreds of people, including high college officials, Nobel laureate scientists, powerful senior professors and the young John Maynard Keynes.[7]

The Sociological Society, which Galton addressed in 1904, was also interested in eugenics because of its scientific aura. Other supporters included Havelock Ellis, George Bernard Shaw, H. G. Wells and Beatrice and Sidney Webb. Indeed, eugenics was widely supported by Marxists, Fabians and feminists. Their emphasis on the collective good and their belief in meritocracy fitted with the eugenic ideology of the time. Paul quotes Sidney Webb: 'No consistent eugenicist can be a "Laisser Faire" individualist unless he throws up the game in despair: He must interfere, interfere, interfere!'[8] Politicians who were members of the Society included A. J. Balfour and Neville Chamberlain, both Prime Ministers (thirty years apart). Other prominent members of the birth control movement, such as Marie Stopes, were also supporters of eugenics. Indeed, Marie Stopes was a eugenicist long before she was an advocate of birth control. It was her eugenic convictions, rather than her interest in compatible sexuality, that spurred her efforts in this direction. As Soloway has noted: 'her particular efforts to provide birth control for the poor had far more to do with her eugenic concerns about the impending "racial darkness" that the adoption of contraception promised to illuminate'.[9]

Inspired by the British movement, various eugenics groups were also established in the USA, such as the Galton Society and the Race Betterment Foundation. These were drawn together under the banner of the American Eugenics Society in 1923. Although smaller than its British equivalent, the American Society had a considerably larger budget, with contributors including luminaries such as John D. Rockefeller. The membership in the USA mirrored its British counterpart, with a predominance of middle-class professionals such as physicians, social workers, clerics and academics. Although most of the members were conservative, others were radical, as in the British movement. As Paul notes, in Georgia, advocates of the New Deal who campaigned for old age pensions, free schoolbooks and well baby clinics also supported eugenic sterilization. Margaret Sanger, the American feminist campaigner for birth control, supported eugenics like her British equivalent, Marie Stopes. Even Helen Keller, the famous blind and deaf campaigner, believed that the objective science of eugenics could be applied to aid decision making about which mentally impaired infants should be eliminated at birth.

An International Eugenic Congress was held in London in 1912. Kevles lists some of the sponsoring vice-presidents as Winston Churchill and Alexander Graham Bell, who called for deaf marriages to be prevented on eugenic grounds. In Britain and in the USA, and increasingly throughout Europe, eugenics was an establishment strategy.

The Eugenics Education Society (renamed the Eugenics Society in 1926) and the American Eugenics Society, alongside the broader eugenic movements, aimed to popularize the scientific messages of eugenics. Although eugenicists disagreed about the strategies for improving the population, they all thought that reproductive decisions were not just personal matters but involved social responsibilities. They conducted lecture tours and produced pamphlets, books and other written material, and films. Eugenic material could also be found at exhibitions and fairs. Kevles quotes the 1910 edition of the *Encyclopaedia Britannica*, which stated that eugenics foresaw 'the organic betterment of the race through the wise application of the laws of heredity'.[10] He also notes that the July 1913 issue of *Cosmopolitan* included an article where the author celebrated eugenics and warned, 'do not marry into a family that carries a defect of the kind that is carried also in your own family strain'.[11] As Allen has shown,[12] the number of articles on eugenics in American periodicals and magazines like *Good Housekeeping* increased more than ten times between 1910 and 1915 and W. E. Castle's popular textbook *Genetics and*

Eugenics went through three editions. *The Science of Life*, a eugenic film, was also distributed by the American Public Health Service between 1922 and 1937. Pernick describes its contents:

> *The Science of Life* emphasised stark mechanical images. It urged 'THE WOMEN OF TOMORROW' to develop strength and beauty through vigorous exercise . . . [It] promised that both 'health and success' awaited the visually attractive [like the *Black Stork*, which dramatised the child murders of Dr Harry Haiselden], couples who illustrate 'wise mating' wear tastefully conservative but up-to-date business suits and dresses on their prosperously stout bodies. Portraying 'others' as ugly was central to labelling them defective, whilst diagnosing 'others' as diseased reinforced the perception of them as repulsive.[13]

Haiselden's euthanasia of 'defective children' gained accolades from the likes of Charles Davenport and Irving Fisher, despite their later efforts to distance themselves from these practices.

British positive eugenic campaigns sought to encourage the middle classes to breed through tax concessions or grants. MacKenzie tells how eugenicists also advocated a stratified education system, to preserve and enhance the status of the genetically superior professional middle classes. More generally, the British Eugenics Society was ambivalent about birth control as a means to prevent the unfit from breeding, because of fears that the middle classes would be the principal users of contraceptives and birth control could therefore have dysgenic consequences. Like the British movement, the American Eugenics Society also encouraged the genetically fit to breed. The Society promoted Better Babies competitions and Fitter Families contests at state fairs as part of this campaign.[14]

One of the most successful British eugenics campaigns concerned the threat of the feeble-minded. This was stimulated by the report of the 1908 Royal Commission on the Care and Control of the Feebleminded, the government's response to concerns about the links between mental and moral deficiency. The Eugenics Society campaigned for legislation to ensure the segregation of the feeble-minded. The 1913 Mental Deficiency Act was hailed as a great victory. This period marked the high point of British eugenicists' success.

In the USA, eugenicists were more successful still, instituting a widespread sterilization programme of inmates of prisons and mental institutions. To surgeons, prison doctors and social reformers alike, the new surgical procedure of vasectomy seemed a simple solution to the growing prison population. Harry Laughlin, the administrator of the Eugenics Record Office, led the sterilization campaign. The aim was to secure legislation that would allow for the compulsory sterilization of inmates of mental institutions, persistent sex offenders, the feeble-minded, moral degenerates and epileptics. By 1935, 26 states had such laws on their books and another ten were waiting to finalize them. Paul notes various surveys that showed considerable public support for these practices. Geneticists too were often supportive, despite the knowledge that the procedure would not meet the eugenic aim of altering the genetic fitness of the population (because of recessive genes). The unsuitability of the unfit to be parents now justified such practices.

The American eugenics movement was also more preoccupied with race than its British counterpart. For example, as Allen notes, Madison Grant's *The Passing of the Great Race* (1916) suggested that the races could be ranked in an 'ethnic pyramid'. A similar theory of racial hierarchy combined with a belief in widespread degeneracy amongst the lower classes also led Laughlin to campaign actively for the Johnston Act (1924) that restricted immigration. As Allen records, Laughlin argued before Congress that 'Making all logical allowances for environmental conditions, which may be unfavourable to the immigrant, the recent immigrants, as a whole, present a higher percentage of inborn socially inadequate qualities than do the older stock.'[15] Despite the critical testimony of geneticist Herbert Spencer Jennings, by that time a strong opponent of eugenics, Allen notes that the Johnston Act passed with considerable majorities in both houses.

Sterilization never became compulsory in the UK. The British eugenics movement was always somewhat cautious about sterilization because of fears of controversy and concerns about it causing the spread of venereal disease. But it did favour voluntary sterilization. A Committee for Legalising Eugenic Sterilization was set up by the Eugenics Education Society in 1929. This committee eventually dissolved into a bigger grouping – the Joint Committee on Voluntary Sterilization – that included representatives from groups such as the Mental Hospitals Association and the Central Association for Mental Welfare. It was this committee that drafted a Sterilization Bill, following the government's Report of the Departmental Committee on Sterilization (the Brock Report) in 1934, which recommended voluntary sterilization. Groups passing resolutions in support of voluntary sterilization included the Royal College of Nursing and several societies for the welfare of the blind. As Mazumdar notes in *Eugenics, Human Genetics and Human Failings*, about half of these were women's groups. There was also apparently considerable public support for the Brock recommendations. As Thomson notes, a *Morning Post* poll at the time claimed that 78.7 per cent of the population were in favour of sterilization (although he observes that opinion polls in this period were not always reliable). However, eugenicists were unable to maintain the momentum in support of voluntary sterilization as the popularity of eugenics waned. The 1937 bill that they supported was not implemented.

The Labour Party, trade unions, the Catholic Church and the British Medical Association all condemned eugenic sterilization proposals, as did the new breed of geneticists, like Lionel Penrose. Eugenics became increasingly associated with the far right. However, in practice, throughout the 1930s some birth control clinics did advocate sterilization, particularly for disabled and working-class women. Thomson gives the example of the Leicestershire National Health Insurance Committee, who advised individuals who were likely to pass on a hereditary disease to be sterilized (at an independent hospital). He also notes that abortion was sometimes justified on eugenic grounds. Trombley notes in *The Right to Reproduce*: 'It had long been Havelock Ellis's view that the whole project of a sterilization bill was dangerous because it merely raised doubts in the minds of doctors who were sterilizing people anyway.'[16]

Eugenic legislation and practices: institutionalization and sterilization

The experiences of people who were violated or imprisoned during this period in the name of eugenics are now beginning to come to wider public attention. Placing these testimonies in the context of eugenic legislation, we now go on to consider institutionalization in the UK and compulsory sterilization in the USA. However, we emphasize once again that a clear boundary between these practices is overly simplistic: institutionalization and sterilization occurred in both countries.

Thomson shows that, at the turn of the century in Britain, the 'feeble-minded', deaf, 'dumb' and blind were all educated in a similar manner. The Elementary Education (Blind and Deaf Children) Act of 1893 had already enshrined the rights of blind and deaf children to elementary education in special day schools run by local authorities, or private residential institutions. The 1902 Education Act went further, leading to the establishment of training colleges and grammar schools for the blind and deaf. Schools or special classes for the feeble-minded were also in existence. And many leading figures in the educational establishment wanted to go further still. Prichard quotes Dr Francis Warner, whose study of 50,000 London schoolchildren was published in 1893. In it he concluded that children who had 'imperfections in bodily development and physiognomy, abnormal neurological responses, poor physical condition due to lack of adequate nutrition or chronic illness and mental dullness' should receive special education.[17]

Special education was justified by appeals to the rights of these children to education despite their disabilities, and their need for special education tailored to their needs, which mainstream education could not provide. But eugenic ideology also played a part in their segregation. Fears that the children's disabilities might affect so-called normal children underlined the need for special schools. And the manner of segregation undermined the rhetoric of special needs. Children with different disabilities were often grouped together, apart from their non-disabled peers. Even physically and mentally disabled children were grouped together and treated similarly.

Institutionalization of the feeble-minded was also fuelled by increasing levels of school inspection. This revealed large numbers of ill and undernourished children, adding to alarm about the national physique. Galton's studies of the inheritance of ability and IQ furthered this sense of pessimism about the prospects of the feeble-minded. Managers of workhouses, prisons and reformatories complained about the disruptive behaviour of the feeble-minded and raised concerns about the vulnerability of feeble-minded girls to sexual advances.

The Royal Commission on the Care and Control of the Feebleminded was established in 1908 in response to these concerns. The report favoured segregated residential homes based on the colony model, pioneered by Mary Dendy and Henry Ashby. The Mental Deficiency Act followed the report in 1913. Although it rejected many of the recommendations of the Commission, it did make allowances for the education of children, deemed by local authorities to be incapable of being educated in special schools, to be passed over to the mental deficiency committees and sent to mental defective schools. In practice, many children remained in special schools, although Prichard notes that by the outbreak of the Second World War, 17,000 children were at mental defective schools.[18]

Potts and Fido have collected the testimonies of inmates of one colony for the feeble-minded in their book *A Fit Person to be Removed*. 'The Park' opened in 1920 to cater for 'the imbecile and idiot class of defectives who in many cases suffer from epilepsy and physical infirmity'.[19] The residents were housed in large villas, segregated by sex and grade of deficiency. They were issued with uniforms and cut off from visitors. Physical punishment was administered, even for incontinence. More able residents were also put to work, including the care of less able residents. As Potts and Fido note, the inmates' medical records show that mental deficiency was widely defined. Frequent mention was made of the children's propensity to cry as confirmation of their diagnosis. Even smiling could be viewed as evidence of defectiveness. One resident, Ernest, was certified following a long period of hospitalization as a result of his congenital impairment, because he was considered to be intellectually underdeveloped. Another, Margaret, had cerebral palsy and at the age of four it was concluded that she would not benefit from education.

Similar institutions were established in the USA. But the practice of compulsory sterilization had a major impact on the numbers therein. Sterilization became a favoured solution to rising costs as pessimism about the prospects of curing defectives grew. Initially it occurred on an ad-hoc basis. One of the first instances of sterilization was in 1898, in the Kansas State Institution for Feeble-Minded Children. Trombley writes of Dr F. Hoyt Pilcher, who was inspired by Herbert Spencer's theory of acquired characteristics (which held that acquired defects could be passed on to the next generation), and who experimented with castration and sterilisation of the inmates. He sterilized 44 boys and 14 girls. Dr Harry Sharp of the Indiana State Reformatory also sterilized nearly 500 males between 1899 and 1907. Paul notes that it was Sharp who helped to persuade the Indiana State legislature to enact the first sterilization law in 1907, which authorized the compulsory sterilization of 'criminals, idiots, rapists and imbeciles'.[20] By 1912 there were sterilization laws in eight states. Although various challenges to this type of legislation occurred, the 1927 case of *Buck* v. *Bell*, which upheld the Virginia law, saw the beginnings of more widespread sterilization. In all, 30 American states had sterilization laws, and the number of victims had reached 60,000 by the 1960s.

Kevles draws attention to Jacob H. Landman's study of sterilization laws in the USA, where he found that sexual offences or moral degeneracy featured prominently in the reasons for sterilization. For example, in California, three-quarters of women who were sterilized were labelled sexually delinquent. There was clearly an emphasis on punishment in these laws and practices, but eugenics still played an important role. Sterilizing sexual delinquents ensured they would not breed. Kevles also notes that because sterilization laws were directed at public institutions it was the lower classes and ethnic minorities who were most affected, as they constituted the bulk of the inmates.

The decline of sterilization programmes in the USA occurred as the atrocities of the Second World War came to widespread attention and Catholics in particular organized to oppose further laws and prevent the implementation of those already on the statute books. But, as we will shortly discuss, sterilization continued in the guise of voluntarism well into the 1970s, in the USA, Scandinavia and Canada. It would also be wrong to think of American or British eugenicists as being naïve about Nazi practices, as we shall go on to discuss in Chapter 3.

Conclusion

This brief historical review has highlighted the different guises that eugenics can take, from an emphasis on compulsory sterilization or euthanasia of the unfit to more benign efforts to encourage the middle classes to breed. We have also shown the diverse groups who were attracted to eugenic ideology, including those from both ends of the political spectrum, and people from a variety of professions, including the sciences and medicine. This chapter has demonstrated that eugenics cannot simply be dismissed as pseudo-science, as its beginnings are intimately tied to the emerging sciences of genetics and psychology in particular. Indeed, some geneticists often led eugenic campaigns (just as other geneticists sometimes led the opposition). There were clearly a variety of class and professional interests at stake, in addition to racist and imperialist ideologies.

It is perhaps ironic that during this period of professionalization, physicians and scientists were honing their categories of disability on the one hand, and leading the eugenic campaign that actually homogenized disabled people on the other. Physically and mentally disabled people, criminals and other stigmatized groups, such as alcoholics and the promiscuous, shared a common status: genetic outsiders. Their visibility amongst the poor and dispossessed exacerbated their victimization, and their incarceration made them prime subjects for study as well as experiment and violation.

But it is not just the scientific and medical professions who should be singled out for criticism, given the investment of the middle classes more generally in eugenic ideology (and indeed science). It is both depressing and instructive to learn that the great reformers whom we hold in such high esteem were so often standard bearers for such thoroughly repugnant views and practices. Too many feminist and socialists showed little solidarity with the disabled, the poor and the socially stigmatised for their example to be treated with reverence. Instead their project was one of control and containment, lest the masses and the deviant should further pollute the new society they were forging.

It is also important to stress that there were important sections of the scientific and genetics professions who resisted the barbarism conducted in their name. While we must note the belated and quiet nature of many of their protests, we acknowledge their role in challenging these more virulent forms of eugenics. However, geneticists and their medical allies forged a new form of eugenics, which Kevles calls reform eugenics, that is perhaps all the more dangerous because of its acceptable face. Before discussing this new phenomenon, we look at those countries that went furthest in implementing eugenic philosophy: Nazi Germany and social democratic Scandinavia.

3

Nazi racial science

In common with Britain, the USA and other European countries, Darwinian ideas had had a great impact in Germany in the late nineteenth and early twentieth centuries. But an explosive mixture of professional, socioeconomic and political factors were to lead to the establishment of a large-scale programme for sterilization, euthanasia and ultimately genocide. Although there is widespread awareness of the Jewish Holocaust, considerably less has been written about the murder of disabled people in Nazi Germany. In this chapter we discuss the development of Nazi racial science and the route to the Holocaust, drawing on several key texts: Michael Burleigh's *Death and Deliverance: 'Euthanasia' in Germany 1900–1945*, and *Ethics and Extermination: Reflections on Nazi genocide*; Henry Friedlander's *The Origins of Nazi Genocide: From euthanasia to the Final Solution* and Hugh Gallagher's *By Trust Betrayed: Patients, physicians and the licence to kill in the Third Reich*.

Intellectual climate

At the turn of the nineteenth century, social Darwinism was popular throughout Europe, Germany being no exception. People were defined according to their biological characteristics in the developing 'science' of racial hygiene. Darwin's theory about the 'survival of the fittest' was used to justify elitism and condemn welfare measures, which were seen as undermining the workings of natural selection. When the German biologist Ernst Haeckel published *The Riddle of the Universe* in 1899, it rapidly became a best seller. The book reinforced the social Darwinian belief that many common impairments and disorders were inherited, not acquired, including conditions such as schizophrenia, depression, paralysis and epilepsy. However, Haeckel went further in arguing that society was not 'bound under all circumstances to maintain and prolong life even when it becomes utterly useless', and he recommended the appointment of a commission to determine who should live and who should die.

In the early twentieth century, the German eugenics movement was just a more unified version of its American equivalent. As Friedlander argues,

> By the scientific standards of the time, eugenic research was on the cutting edge of science. Its practitioners were respected scholars from various scientific disciplines who occupied important positions in major universities and published their results in major scholarly journals. Their research tools were the most advanced available at the time, and they prided themselves on applying them meticulously. Their failing was not methodological error but their inability to recognise the ways in which their own prejudices corrupted their premises and tainted their conclusions.[1]

The German Society for Race Hygiene won support from all political parties, including the Social Democrats. For example, Social Democrat Alfred Grotjahn, Professor of Social Hygiene at University of Berlin, advocated sterilization of the unfit, while Social Democrat leader Karl Kautsky opposed leaving abortion decisions to individual women as 'unsocialist'. However, the efforts of the race hygienists mainly centred on positive eugenics until the defeat of Germany in the First World War.

The experience of defeat radicalized the German professional classes, many of whom turned to extreme nationalism. Often, eugenicists later became Nazi supporters: for example, Fritz Lenz, Professor of Racial Hygiene at Berlin. A split developed between eugenicists who supported the racial superiority of Nordic and German peoples and others who did not take a racial view. From then on, the Aryan supremacy ideas were increasingly dominant, to be followed later on by growing anti-semitism. By 1932, there were more than 40 courses on race hygiene at German universities.

The First World War also had a terrible impact on the German psychiatric system. Vast numbers of psychiatric patients died during the conflict from hunger, disease and neglect. Burleigh quotes studies estimating that approximately 30 per cent of the asylum population died between 1914 and 1919.[2] Another consequence of the war was the use of dehumanizing treatment of exhausted or 'neurotic' soldiers through shock therapies. However, positive and liberal changes to German psychiatry also followed in the post-war period, which included an increased emphasis on the community, rather than the asylum, and the development of occupational therapy techniques within the institutions.

Burleigh suggests that both reforms had two dangerous side-effects.

The first brought the wider population of abnormal and deviant people to the attention of psychiatrists, a discovery that led to the fashion for cataloguing mental degeneracy in genealogical form, and a certain pessimism about the possibility for cure or progress. The second enabled many patients to play a productive role within the institution, but also highlighted the residuum of people who were too impaired to make any economic contribution. Similarly, as psychiatry developed new drugs and techniques in the 1930s, success with some patients made the contrast with incurable cases more acute. Long before the Nazis came to power, some psychiatrists were suggesting that this sub-class of psychiatric patients might be killed.

Burleigh notes that in 1920 Karl Binding, a lawyer, and Alfred Hoche, a psychiatrist, had written a book called *The Permission to Destroy Life Unworthy of Life* which had challenged values such as the 'sanctity of human life' and emotions such as 'pity', and had emphasized, instead, the economic burden of disabled people, proposing 'mercy killing' as the solution. Their argument started with the idea that suicide was a human right, which should not be unlawful. Having established the benefits of voluntary euthanasia in the case of terminal illness, Binding went on to justify the non-consensual killing of mentally deficient or mentally ill people. The book suggested that whether life is worth living depended not only on its worth to the individual, but also on its worth to society. Hoche argued that the lives of the 'incurably feeble minded' were 'without purpose': as mere 'human ballast', they imposed a 'terribly difficult burden' on relatives and society. Moreover, the wartime sacrifices of healthy people meant that sacrifice of 'valueless' people could be justified: the alternative was the use of national resources for non-productive purposes.

Various practical measures of euthanasia were proposed, including the necessary protection of doctors against the outcry of relatives, and the side-benefit that killing of defectives would bring to research, particularly brain research. In conclusion, Binding discussed the procedures that would be necessary for implementing 'mercy killing', including an authorization committee of jurist and physicians. Of course, it was still possible that some errors of judgement would be made but, he concluded, 'humanity loses due to error so many members, that one more or less really does not make a difference'.

These were not unpopular or extreme opinions in 1920s Germany. Ewald Meltzer was director of the Katherinenhof asylum for backward juveniles, and a passionate critic of Binding and Hoche. However, Michael Burleigh notes that when Meltzer surveyed parents of his residents in 1925, he was shocked to discover that 73 per cent of respondents said they would approve the 'painless curtailment' of the life of their children, if experts had established that they were suffering from 'incurable idiocy'. Furthermore, half of those who disapproved of this were prepared to countenance such euthanasia in the event that the child was orphaned. These responses were frequently quoted in Nazi propaganda.

The rise of the Nazis

A key element in the rise to power of the Nazis was the appalling economic conditions experienced by Germans after their defeat in the First World War. Industrial destruction, the heavy reparations imposed after the Treaty of Versailles and the worldwide economic depression of the 1930s created insecurity, instability and suffering throughout Germany. In this context, arguments about the economic burden of disabled people carried particular weight. Justifications for racial hygiene and eugenics often depended on the need to save resources and space. Care for disabled people was seen as a waste of money. Hugh Gallagher shows that these ideas were even enshrined in the maths books that were used in schools after the Nazis came to power, with questions such as: 'If the building of a lunatic asylum costs six million marks and it costs fifteen thousand marks to build each house on a housing estate, how many of the latter could be built for the price of one asylum?'

An early consequence of the Nazi regime was the withdrawal of resources from institutions. More people were crammed into asylums. As a consequence, the doctor–patient ratio deteriorated: in some institutions, there were as many as 500 patients to one doctor, whereas previously there had been around 160. The amounts spent on food for patients were cut. This was at a time when the economy was actually improving. Many psychiatrists had become Nazi supporters, and many unsuitable people entered nursing to avoid unemployment.

Of course, Hitler himself took a social Darwinist view, stating that 'the strongest asserts its will; it is the law of nature' and that 'Nature is cruel, therefore we are also entitled to be cruel.' He wrote in admiration of Sparta, claiming that 'The exposure of the sick, weak, deformed children, in short their destruction, was more decent and in truth a thousand times more humane than the wretched insanity of our day which seeks to preserve the most pathological subjects.' Along with obsessive concern about the biological basis of the German race and the threat of 'mongrelization', *Mein Kampf* was full of prejudice against disabled people, and the need to prevent their reproduction. Hitler's views in this area were reflected by wider German society: in the 1920s and 1930s, there was a widespread view that it was shameful to be disabled.

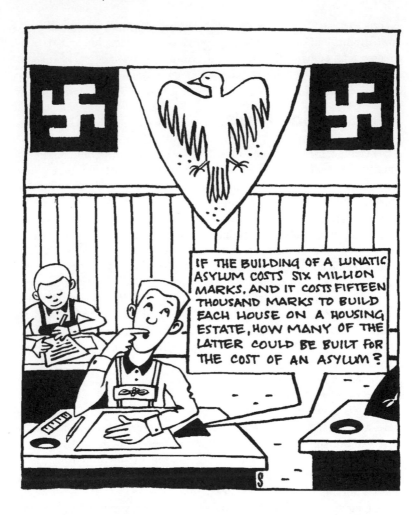

The popular media were full of these messages. Hugh Gallagher describes how contemporary films promoted prejudice against disabled people, labelled 'useless eaters' or 'life unworthy of life'. People with learning difficulties or mental health problems were dehumanized, and often lumped together with criminals and murderers. In these films and books, Jews were often represented as being particularly prone to physical or mental degeneracy.

One of Gallagher's examples of the reinforcement of eugenic ideology in mass culture is the film *I Accuse*, which centred on a husband murdering a wife who had multiple sclerosis. Adapted from a pro-euthanasia novel by the ophthalmologist Helmut Unger (*Sendung und Gewissen*), it won an award at the Venice Biennale. Unger was later a member of the group that planned the children's euthanasia programme.

Michael Burleigh describes how the advent of Nazi government in 1933 meant that asylums became freakshows. Between 1933 and 1939, 21,000 people visited the Eglfing-Haar institution, including 6,000 members of the Schutzstaffel (SS), some of whom advocated setting up machine guns to mow down the residents. Nazi periodicals openly advocated killing the mentally ill. The cult of strength and youth had little time for people who were elderly, frail or disabled.

Sterilization

Eugenic propaganda became eugenic practice after the accession of the Nazis to power. The Law for the Prevention of Genetically Impaired Progeny was implemented on 14 July 1933. It stated that 'any person suffering from a hereditary disease may be rendered incapable of begetting children by means of a surgical operation, provided it is established by a scientific medical experience as very highly probable that any children he might beget would inherit some serious physical or mental defect'. A contemporary report of the American Neurological Association shows the extent to which this law reflected mainstream eugenic theory:

> It is fair to state that the Sterilization Act is not a product of Hitler's regime in that its main tenets were proposed and considered several years earlier before the Nazi regime took possession of Germany. There is no doubt that the Act conforms closely with the present knowledge of medical eugenics.

Indeed, enthusiasm for the Sterilization Act was being expressed in the *American Journal of Psychiatry* as late as July 1942.

Between 14 July 1933 and 1 September 1939, the Nazi regime sterilized approximately 375,000 people, on the grounds of a range of heritable conditions. The following list, taken from Hugh Gallagher's *By Trust Betrayed*, enumerates these criteria, the figure in brackets being the percentage sterilized under this heading in the year 1934.

1. Congenital feeble-mindedness (52.9%)
2. Schizophrenia (25.4%)
3. Folie circulaire (manic depressive psychosis) (3.2%)
4. Hereditary epilepsy (14%)
5. Hereditary St Vitus Dance (Huntington's) (0.2%)

6.   Hereditary blindness (0.6%)
7.   Hereditary deafness (1%)
8.   Severe hereditary physical deformity (0.3%)
9.   Severe alcoholism on a discretionary basis (2.4%)

Despite these apparently 'scientific' categories, the notion of heritability was often arbitrary. For example, originally only 'congenital schizophrenia' was included, but the category was expanded to cover all incidences of this condition. The category 'alcoholism' is obviously subjective, and even recovering alcoholics were likely to be included. On the other hand, haemophilia, an obvious congenital condition, was not listed.

Perhaps the vaguest criterion, however, was feeble-mindedness. The process for compulsory sterilization involved hereditary health courts, secret tribunals run by doctors. Henry Friedlander notes that examiners were to administer an oral test to people suspected of feeble-mindedness. Questions included: Who was Luther? Who discovered America? When is Christmas? What is the capital of France? However, even if the subject passed the test, they were still vulnerable. The subjective judgement of the medical examiner was equally important: it was possible to answer the questions correctly and still be sent for sterilization, if the candidate's appearance and behaviour suggested feeble-mindedness.[3]

In fact, all the historians describe how doctors played a central role in the whole process. Three-quarters of all denunciations of people to the health courts came from the medical profession. Contemporary reports show that the public health service and the medical profession clamoured for sterilization even when the hereditary health courts had turned down a particular application. Other professionals also played a role in weeding out the unfit: school teachers were encouraged to set their pupils the task of constructing their family trees, in order to identify any defective members, while mayors reported single mothers to the courts.

Sterilization had a terrible impact on the German population, 5 per cent of whom underwent the operation. In the post-war Hollywood film *Judgement at Nuremberg*, Montgomery Clift has a moving cameo role as a man with learning difficulties who had been sterilized: his testimony is incoherent, but the haunting look in his eyes conveys the human cost of the eugenic policy. In a real-life example of the irrationality and cruelty of the measure, a workman in Saxony who had lost his leg in an accident was said to have a diminished earning capacity. He was sterilized against his will. As a result of this trauma, he later committed suicide.

Shame and humiliation were not the only consequences of the operation, which could sometimes result in the death of the victim. While approximately equal numbers of men and women were sterilized, many more women than men died as a direct result of the procedure. For these reasons, there was a high level of resistance to what had been nicknamed 'the Hitler cut': 37.3 per cent of victims gave approval and 24.1 per cent had approval given by legal guardians, while 38.6 per cent were forced to submit.[4]

The sterilization policy marked the full application of eugenic principles. However, the regime did not stop there. Following the Nuremberg Laws, the Marriage Health Law of September 1935 prohibited marriage if either party suffered from mental derangement, a hereditary disease or a contagious illness such as tuberculosis or venereal disease. Couples required a Marriage Fitness Certificate from their Public Health Office before being allowed to marry. Given that people with congenital conditions had probably already been sterilized, this measure seems superfluous, even from a eugenic point of view. It demonstrates that the regime was obsessed with eliminating 'defectives', not just for the future, but also in the present. As Henry Friedlander has argued, 'Although the murder of handicapped adults was both unnecessary and senseless because they were already sterilised and thus unable to produce descendants, for the killers a logical progression led from exclusion to extermination.'[5] First the Nazis prevented the birth of more disabled people. Then they killed disabled children. Finally, they killed disabled adults.

Euthanasia

While Nazi propaganda had long espoused the need for 'mercy killing', requests from relatives of disabled people, received by the Chancellery of the Führer, contributed to the decision to implement euthanasia. Hitler had previously suggested that the advent of war would be the best time to implement the policy. The turning point was the Knauer case in early 1939, which involved a child born blind and with missing limbs in Leipzig. After the child's father wrote to Hitler asking for euthanasia, the Führer's personal physician, Karl Brandt, was dispatched to inspect the baby and authorize the killing.

The adult euthanasia programme began on September 1939. It originated in a personal order of Adolf Hitler on private stationery. Stamped 'top secret', it read:

> Reichsleiter Bouhler and Dr Med. Brandt are charged with responsibility to extend the powers of specific doctors in such a way that, after the most careful assessment of their condition, those suffering from illnesses deemed to be incurable may be granted a mercy death.[6]

This was never a formal law or government order. Later, this was to cause problems with relatives and judges, many of whom were concerned less about the practice of killing disabled people than about the fact that this was against the law of the time. However, Hitler was probably aware that the policy would cause considerable opposition at home and abroad, and always resisted pressure to legalize euthanasia. For the same reason, a separate and secret department within the Führer's own Chancellery was set up to implement the programme.

The new organization was based in a confiscated Jewish villa at number 4, Tiergartenstrasse, hence it was known as T-4. Philipp Bouhler directed the T-4 programme, while SS Colonel Viktor Brack was in charge of day-to-day administration, assisted by three physicians: Dr Herbert Linden (in charge of sanitoriums and nursing homes in the Ministry of Interior), Professor Dr Werner Heyde (formerly Professor of Psychiatry at the University of Würzburg) and his deputy, Professor Dr Paul Nitsche.

Hugh Gallagher tells how three spurious corporations were set up to handle operations. The Foundation for the Care of Institutions in the Public Interest was responsible for budgetary and financial matters. For example, it collected money for the care of patients from their families, continuing to levy charges even after the disabled person had been killed. The Reich Association of Sanitoriums and Nursing Homes was responsible for administration. Finally, the Charitable Patient Transport Company (known as Gekrat) moved people by van and bus from their institutions to the killing centres. A separate Reich Committee for Research on Hereditary and Constitutional Severe Diseases was responsible for children's euthanasia, but was based at the same address.

A group of leading doctors were invited to a secret meeting in August 1939, where the purpose of the scheme was explained to them, and they were invited to participate, which they all agreed to do.[7] Neither at this point nor at any time was anyone forced to take part in the T-4 programme. The Reich Department of Health issued a decree on 21 September, requiring each regional government area to send a full list of institutions in their locality. Subsequently, questionnaires were sent to each institution asking for details of every resident. These cursory forms included short statements about racial origin, what work the patient could do, what their diagnosis was, and the original cause of the impairment. In the early days, physicians at the institutions, not knowing the purpose of the form, often exaggerated the incapacity of their patients in an attempt to prevent productive people being removed to work for the war effort.

The questionnaires were collected in and reviewed by a panel of about 40 medical experts, which included nine university professors of medicine, whose job was to mark each form with a plus or a minus symbol.

These professionals probably did not regard their acts as killing, but as normal medical practice: they were just involved in the supervision of a new type of therapy. Assessors were paid 10 pfennigs per questionnaire and processed very large numbers of questionnaires – each did tens of thousands.

Subsequently, Heyde, Nitsche and Linden, the 'senior experts', reviewed all the forms. Although they were doctors, they were busy administrating the organization. Their cursory checking of the forms was not a careful safeguard, but a cover to make the process seem scientific and to take responsibility away from the junior panel of experts. From start to finish, the whole process was extremely hurried. As Friedlander suggests, 'the impressive medical edifice constructed by T4 to safeguard against unprofessional evaluation was a façade'.[8]

Patients were selected on grounds of medical condition and level of productivity. Concepts such as 'useless eaters', 'life unworthy of life' and 'human ballast' were now being used to decide who would live and who would die. Patients were selected because of conditions such as schizophrenia, depression, mental retardation, dwarfism, paralysis, epilepsy, sometimes delinquency, perversion, alcoholism and antisocial behaviour. In order to avoid weakening army morale, veterans of the First World War were exempted, but only if they had received medals, or been wounded, or fought with special valour.

Once patients had been selected, lists of names were sent to the T-4 transport office, which organized transport lists in order to maintain a regular flow of patients to killing centres. Institutions were given notification a few days before transfer, and strict instructions as to who was to be collected, and how they were to be presented. For example, patients were to have their names taped to their back between their shoulder blades.

Gallagher describes how Gekrat was staffed by male nurses recruited from the SS. Because they wore white uniforms, but retained their black SS boots, they were known as 'white coat–black boots' by hospital staff. The ominous grey buses took the disabled people to one of six killing centres at Grafeneck, Brandenburg, Hartheim, Sonnenstein, Bernburg and Hadamar, all of which had the official title of State Hospital and Nursing Home. Early experiments, witnessed by many of the T-4 medical personnel, had shown that gassing with carbon monoxide was an efficient killing technique, and gas chambers were rigged up in each centre, disguised as showers. Patients arrived at the centre, many of them very anxious about their fate, and were processed as if it was a normal hospital. Then they were undressed, taken for a 'shower', and filed into the gas chamber. The medical officer in charge of the centre then turned on the gas tap, and the staff waited for ten minutes until all the patients were dead. Orderlies then dragged the bodies out of the gas chambers and took them off to be cremated in nearby ovens. Those patients who had gold dental work had previously been given a special mark on their skin, so that their teeth could be broken off and sent to Berlin. This gold made a valuable contribution to the budget of the T-4 operation.

An elaborate charade was used to disguise the fate of these patients. Families were first notified that their relative had been transferred to another institution. Then the 'receiving institution' (killing centre) sent notification that the person had arrived, but that visits were prohibited. Finally, some time later, the relatives were notified that the patient had unfortunately died, but that due to the danger of epidemics, the body had to be immediately cremated. However, an urn containing the relative's ashes could be obtained on request. Considerable ingenuity was used in the construction of spurious causes of death (there was even talk of having a T-4 national conference to discuss the problem). Typical explanations for sudden death included diagnoses such as brain tumour, abscessed tonsils, appendicitis, septicaemia and pneumonia.

Up to 75 people were gassed at the same time. But as a member of staff from the Hartheim centre, quoted by Friedlander, testified after the war: 'Once 150 persons were gassed at one time. The gas chamber was so full that the people in it could scarcely fall down, and the corpses were therefore so jammed together that we could pry them apart only with great difficulty.' Burning the bodies was more technically difficult than killing them, and was much slower. Often a backlog built up. The 3 kilograms of ash shovelled into the urn that was sent later to relatives was merely a portion of the total residue, rather than being the specific remains of the loved one. Local people noticed the constant smoke and terrible smells. The centres at Brandenburg and Grafeneck had to be closed due to local hostility, which resulted from increasing awareness of what was going on. However, by the time awareness and protest had mounted, leading Hitler to issue an order to stop the T-4 programme in August 1941, at least 70,000 people had been killed.

Children's euthanasia

Killing of disabled children actually commenced before the T-4 programme, and continued after the main programme had been halted. Friedlander notes: 'The children were considered especially crucial because they represented posterity; elimination of those considered diseased and deformed was essential if the eugenic and racial purification program was to succeed.'[9] Prior to the official policy, zealous Nazi doctors like Dr Hermann Pfannmüller at Eglfing-Haar hospital outside Munich had been starving children to death throughout the 1930s. As with adult euthanasia, although bureaucrats organized the scheme, it was ordinary physicians who implemented the killing of disabled children.

The first step of official euthanasia for children came with a decree on 18 August 1939, instructing that all defective newborns and infants under the age of three should be reported. This included children with deformed limbs, head and spinal column; paralysis and palsy; dwarfism; blindness and deafness; and idiocy, Down's syndrome and various brain abnormalities. Although this official order originated in the Ministry of Health, reports were again dealt with by the Chancellery of the Führer, Hitler's private office. A post office box number was provided for replies. These were dealt with by another front organization, the Reich Committee for the Scientific Registration of Serious Hereditary Ailments, which was another occupant of the house at number 4, Tiergartenstrasse. The operation was headed by Hans Hefelmann and Richard von Hegener. Like all those involved in euthanasia, they used pseudonyms to evade responsibility: both men signed themselves as Dr Klein.

The order maintained the pretence of a scientific motive. Friedlander notes that 'early registration of the appropriate cases involving hereditary deformations and mental retardation [was] essential for the clarification of scientific questions'.[10] The sample report form asked for details such as: name, age, sex, description of illness, restriction on child's ability to function, details about hospital stay and name of hospital, projected life expectancy, and chances for improvement. One side of a page was allocated for these answers.

Three doctors – Wentzler, Catel (Chair of Paediatrics at Leipzig) and Heinze – then reviewed the cases and marked the form with a plus or a minus sign. If all three concurred in their judgement, killing went ahead: to use the prevailing euphemism, they issued an 'authorization to treat' the child. The babies and toddlers were transferred to one of 28 killing centres, which were often part of an existing hospital and known as 'specialist children's wards'. There they were killed by lethal injection, or more commonly by overdose of everyday medications administered in cups of tea. These were more easily disguised, especially if the drugs did not kill directly, but led to subsequent death from pneumonia or other medical complications. The police provided the very large numbers of medications that the process needed.

In general, it was easier for the euthanasia bureaucrats to deal with institutionalized children than those who lived with their families. Although some families supported, and even requested, 'mercy killing', others were very reluctant to let their children be taken away. Officials used deception about the possibility of cure on the special wards. Encouragement, pressure and ultimately coercion were applied in order to force parents to co-operate. In theory, the criterion for euthanasia was the presence of an incurable, not necessarily terminal, condition. But the Reich Committee and its physicians (many of whom were very young and inexperienced) did not follow their own rules or observe restraint. Gallagher reports that

> Although at first only the very young were to be included, soon enough the age limit was lifted from three to five – ultimately even teenagers were included. In some places the selection process was turned over to nurses and orderlies. Qualifying social characteristics came to include such things as bed-wetting, pimples, a swarthy complexion, or even annoying the nurses.[11]

There were various changes to the process or the killing techniques: for example, from 7 June 1940, a more extensive questionnaire was used. In some institutions, children were killed by starvation: in Bavaria, this was the official policy adopted from November 1942.

In at least one centre, killing continued even after the end of the war. Friedlander notes that the town of Kaufbeuren was occupied by American troops in April 1945, but the local hospital was not investigated immediately. However, after hearing the rumours circulating, there was an investigation which found that euthanasia was carrying on: four-year-old Richard Jenne, perhaps the last victim of the Nazi euthanasia programme, had died on 29 May. By then, at least 5,000 other children had been killed.

Wild euthanasia

After the official halt of adult euthanasia, random and localized killing of disabled people continued in the 'wild euthanasia' operation. No more gassings were carried out, but the techniques of children's euthanasia – starvation and lethal injection – were adopted on a wide scale throughout Germany. These routine killings took place at Eichberg, Hadamar, Kalmenhof, Mesertiz-Obrawalde and Tiegenhof, among other centres. Murder in hospital was more easily concealed than transport to centralized killing centres: at Mesertiz-Obrawalde up to 10,000 were killed, usually during the middle of night, by drug overdose or lethal injection.

The pool of potential victims of 'wild euthanasia' also expanded to include elderly people and 'antisocial elements'. Foreigners were particularly vulnerable. By 1944, there were many forced labourers from the East in the German Reich who could no longer work due to tuberculosis and other infectious diseases, and who could not be returned home because of the advance of the Red Army; they were simply killed by injections. Hugh Gallagher reports on an anti-tuberculosis programme in occupied Poland that involved physicians riding shotgun across the countryside, shooting peasants who looked tubercular from their cars.

As the war continued, murder became more widespread. Some reports suggest that euthanasia personnel were even used to kill wounded soldiers of the German army on the Eastern Front, for example at Minsk. In the final stages of the war, under Aktion Brandt, mentally ill and long-term care patients were systematically killed, in order to free hospital beds for short-term ill patients from hospitals destroyed by bombing.

From the outbreak of the war, euthanasia was also implemented in the conquered territories to the east of Germany. As the troops invaded, they had been followed by divisions of the SS and other units, who eliminated 'lives unworthy of life' in a ruthless manner. For example, the SS had taken over Pomeranian state hospitals and killed those incurable patients who did not have relatives likely to be concerned. Mentally ill and disabled people were taken to Neustadt in West Prussia, where they were killed in the forest by being shot one by one in the back of the neck, and then buried in mass graves. The SS Eimann Battalion had killed approximately 3,500 patients in the last months of 1939.

Similar methods were used to kill Polish disabled patients. For example, Friedlander describes how German security police shot all 420 patients at the psychiatric hospital of Chelmno, near Lublin, on 12 January 1940. After the invasion of Russia on 22 June 1941, the Einsatzgruppen followed the troops, exterminating Jews, Gypsies and disabled people in the Soviet Union. General Eduard Wagner, quartermaster of the German army, noted in September 1941 that 'Russians consider the feeble-minded holy. Nevertheless, killing necessary.'

Various methods were used to kill these large numbers of people. In Minsk, in the autumn of 1941, the Nazis experimented with dynamiting their victims. Patients were locked into a pillbox that was then exploded. Observers reported the total destruction of both the pillbox and the patients. Parts of bodies were strewn over a wide area, and limbs had to be collected from surrounding trees. Experiments with gas were more successful. Similarly, 100,000 victims were killed at the Kiev Pathological Institute by lethal injection.

From the spring of 1941, the T-4 organization was invited to work in the concentration camps, under a programme known as special treatment 14f13. This involved selected prisoners from all camps administered by the Inspectorate of the Concentration Camps and was a collaboration between T-4 personnel and the SS. T-4 physicians were sent to make final selection of the victims, not because this was a skilled process, but probably in order to ensure the T-4 organization a continuing function. Inspectors used modified T-4 questionnaires, but also focused on Jews and so-called anti-socials. The main criterion for killing was the inability to do physical work. The 'medical inspection' was very cursory: patients filed past physicians sitting at tables who placed a plus or minus on the questionnaire. At Buchenwald, two physicians processed 873 prisoners in five days. Prisoners who were Jewish were not even examined. The victims were then sent to be gassed at the six euthanasia killing centres. Staff did not differentiate camp prisoners from their previous victims, except that the prison uniform was different from the institutional clothing to which they were accustomed.

The 14f13 programme ended in 1943, after up to 20,000 people had been killed. The camps were now exploiting prisoner labour more effectively, and killing in the concentration camps was becoming more ambitious. After this date, Hartheim was the only euthanasia centre that continued in operation. Friedlander notes that the main historical significance of 14f13 was the role it played as a link between euthanasia and the Final Solution. The same techniques – the gas, the extraction of dental gold, the burning of the bodies – that had been pioneered in the killing of disabled people were now applied to the murder of vast numbers of Jewish prisoners. Much of the equipment (gas chambers and gas vans) and about a hundred of the personnel were transferred directly from euthanasia to the Holocaust. As Friedlander concludes: 'The success of the euthanasia policy convinced the Nazi leadership that mass murder was technically feasible, that ordinary men and women were willing to kill large numbers of innocent human beings, and that the bureaucracy would cooperate in such an unprecedented exercise.'[12]

Perpetrators

Gallagher argues:

> Although this program was authorized by Hitler and carried out under the auspices of the National Socialist government of the Third Reich, it would be a mistake to call it a Nazi program. It was not. The program was conceived by physicians and operated by them. They did the killing. While many of these physicians were Nazis, many more were not. The program's sponsors and senior participants were the leading medical professors and psychiatrists of Germany, men of international reputation.[13]

Half of Germany's 15,000 doctors ultimately became members of the Nazi Party. The more enthusiastic had joined the National Socialist German Physicians' League, which beat up Jewish doctors on 1 April 1933, and called for a new medicine on anti-individualist, social Darwinist lines. But doctors generally benefited from the Nazi takeover of power.

Nazi accession brought racial hygiene to the fore, together with the implementation of public health measures. After the instability of the Weimar
period, the professional income and status of doctors rose.

Most doctors co-operated with the eugenics and euthanasia policies of
the Nazis: about 350 were involved directly. According to Gallagher,

> The fact . . . that distinguished professors of medicine and psychiatry
> and quite well-known physicians agreed to participate, and that detailed
> briefings were given not just to medical leaders but to sizable numbers
> of practising doctors, leads to an inescapable conclusion: the medical
> establishment of Germany, leadership and rank and file, raised no very
> significant objections to the program, placed no hindrance to its pur-
> suit.[14]

While some academics have labelled the euthanasia programme 'medical
killing', it was not medicalized in any real sense. Although Hitler had stip-
ulated that doctors had to be involved, there was nothing scientific or
technical about the procedure. As one doctor complained, 'you don't need
a medical degree to turn a gas tap'. The many doctors who were involved
at various stages of the programme were using their power to operate as
professional murderers, not in any clinical capacity.

Gallagher also notes that no one was forced to become involved in the
programme: several individuals declined, and none suffered negative consequences as a result. For example, Dr F. Hölzel declined the invitation to
work in killing units, saying that although he did not oppose euthanasia, he
was himself 'too soft' to implement it. Some doctors actively resisted the
euthanasia programme. After attending the initial T-4 briefing, Professor
Gottfried Ewald, himself a disabled veteran of the First World War, wrote
letters of protest to the authorities: he was ignored, but not punished. Professors Pohlisch and Panse called a secret meeting of physicians in Bonn
to work out a sabotage strategy. For example, the questionnaires could be
faked to show that the individual was working and important to the war
effort. Professor Walter Creutz managed to save 3,000 out of 4,000 people
designated for euthanasia. Other doctors said no to the instructions, took
patients off the Gekrat buses or refused to co-operate.

However, most doctors obeyed laws, followed regulations and ignored
what was happening. Some doctors were enthusiastic Nazis, and others
were committed to the eugenic philosophy. Junior doctors signed up because of the influence of respected senior figures in the profession. Many
would have seen participation as a good career move. They would benefit
from being close to the centre of power, and from good pay and conditions,
and from being exempted from serving on the front line of the war.

Others were able to evade personal guilt by the complex structure of the euthanasia programme, as Gallagher argues. While almost every local physician in Germany was involved in the initial submission of questionnaires, the control of the process was located elsewhere. The bureaucracy ensured that there was no single point of responsibility. The killing decision was extended in time and space between the local doctor, the assessing committee, the review physician, the transportation staff, the killing centre staff and the gas chamber physician. They all did a separate job and were able to convince themselves that they were only following orders, or that they were not personally to blame.

Doctors who were not involved in the programme itself benefited from the opportunities for research that it presented. Several research institutes had close connections with euthanasia and arranged for corpses to be sent for autopsy and analysis. For example, Gallagher tells of Professor Julius Hallervorden from Kaiser Willhelm Institute for Brain Research – now the Max Planck Institute – who received at least 696 brains from institutions and even visited killing centres to perform autopsies. Hallervorden was a very prominent brain disease researcher, distinguished by having Hallervorden-Spatz disease named after him. After the war, he was exonerated from implication in euthanasia by his American psychiatric colleagues. Other centres were sent groups of patients for observation before they were killed and autopsied. These included the research unit at Brandenburg-Görden, headed by Hans Heinze, and the Clinic for Psychiatry and Neurology at Heidelberg, directed by Professor Carl Schneider.

Subsequently, in the concentration camps, various medical experiments were conducted, taking advantage of the relaxation of normal research ethics. No consent was needed, nor any regard for the welfare of the subjects. Some directly involved the death of the patient, for example in the testing of the effects of low pressure at high altitude, or of hypothermia. Vaccines were tested at Buchenwald and Natzweiler, and methods of treating combat wounds investigated at Ravensbrück. There were also research projects on methods of sterilizing rapidly and preferably covertly, using injections or high doses of X-rays. Much of the scientific methodology and many of the aims of this research were legitimate, although it was all totally barbarous and unethical.

By contrast, the notorious Joseph Mengele offers an example of obsessive and unscientific research. He gained doctorates in physical anthropology and medicine and developed an interest in the genetic study of twins and families. He wanted to pursue research into 'racial hygiene'. After the Nazi takeover, he joined the SS. In 1943–4 he was a physician at the Auschwitz-Birkenau concentration camp. Free of ethical or legal restrictions, he was able to use it as his personal research laboratory, using imprisoned Jewish physicians to conduct research, and other inmates as subjects. Among his macabre interests was an obsession with eye colour: he collected pairs of eyes that were differently coloured, to see if he could find ways of changing eye colour. He was also interested in dwarfs, Gypsies and particularly twins.

Gallagher also describes how, as well as doctors, a whole range of ordinary bureaucrats and functionaries were involved. Most of these managers had joined the Nazis in their twenties, before the seizure of power; many were members of the Sturm Abteilung (SA) and the SS. They were loyal and efficient managers, who had willingly joined the operation. These were more than just desk-bound killers: all had observed the killings directly and were involved in the execution as well as the planning of euthanasia. For example, they arranged the supply of gas from the IG Farben company, or the shipments of poisons. T-4 itself needed staff, from builders, administrators, drivers and stokers, to the metal workers employed on stamping out the little plaques on each urn of ashes. It was a very ordinary, if highly secretive, governmental organization. For example, it had its own statistician, who worked out that 70,273 'disinfections' saved the Reich 885,439,980 marks over a period of ten years, and that Germany had been saved 13,492,440 kilograms of meat and wurst. With a few exceptions, most of these employees were not thugs, psychopaths or fanatics: they were ordinary people.

Gallagher notes that, in society at large, one group of professionals who became aware of what was going on were the lawyers. The judiciary had not known about euthanasia, which was illegal. They learned about the programme in various ways: for example, people who were wards of court disappeared suddenly after being transferred to certain institutions. State prosecutors needed to track down people who had committed crimes but were committed to state hospitals as being mentally incapable: often they were required as witnesses or defendants, but were unable to be located. There were also many rumours, and protests from relatives.

There were various appeals to Franz Gürtner, the Reich Minister for Justice. Initially, the ministry started collating all the information. Then Pastor Braune, who had become a one-person campaign against the disappearances, had a private meeting with Gürtner. By late July 1940, the minister was forced to complain to the Chancellery of the Führer. The judiciary were being put in an impossible position by the killings: they demanded either an end to the illegal programme or the promulgation of a law to regularize it. Gallagher suggests:

> It is not unfair to say that throughout the legal community there developed a strong desire to have the killing codified. The concern expressed

in letter after letter is not that the killing be stopped, but that proper legal procedures according to law be established so that the killing could proceed in a proper and organised manner.[15]

Eventually, on 27 August, Bouhler sent Gürtner a copy of Hitler's order.

The Justice Minister realized that this order did not have the force of law, but he was unable to do anything about it: Hitler had adamantly refused to formalize the policy, despite various attempts to draft a statute. The ministry therefore instructed regional attorneys general to allow the investigations to lapse. From then on, the Justice Ministry collaborated closely with the Chancellery of the Führer to avoid blunders and to co-ordinate the killing. Eventually, a meeting was held on 23 and 24 April 1941, where all the leaders of the judiciary were given a full briefing about the T-4 programme, and instructed on how to respond officially. The legal authorities had moved from passive co-operation to active collaboration.

Banality of evil

The memorable phrase 'the banality of evil', first coined by Hannah Arendt, comes to mind when we read about the details of the Nazi extermination systems. The practicalities of the T-4 programme were particularly gruesome, showing the extent to which ordinary people could become inured to brutality. The staff were recruited at random and gained experience on the job, but they soon became capable of extreme callousness and inhumanity. For example, nurses and doctors were given bonuses for taking part in the programme. All T-4 employees were eligible for cut-price dental work, using gold taken from the mouths of the victims.

There are also reports of medical experts, on tours of inspection of the killing centres, turning the trips into opportunities for gastronomic delights or, conversely, complaining at the poor quality of food and accommodation on offer. Many centres gained reputations for drunkenness and sexual excess. Burleigh reports that 'In some centres (notoriously the Kalmenhof at Idstein), the tensions of the job were soothed by a visit to the wine cellars to mark every fiftieth killing with copious amounts of wine and cider.'[16] In another macabre episode, there was a celebration at Hadamar, after the ten thousandth victim had been killed: the body was cremated in a special ceremony, where the staff dressed up and were harangued in mystical tones by the centre director.

As Michael Burleigh explains, bureaucratic errors were an inevitable consequence of such an enormous and secretive programme. For example, one family received two urns of ashes after their relative died. In another case, next of kin were informed of the death of a woman who was still alive and healthy in an institution. Causes of death were sometimes obviously erroneous: for example, appendicitis might be indicated as a cause of death in a person who had had their appendix removed ten years previously. On one occasion, two people of the same name were confused, and the wrong one was taken to be killed. When the error was revealed, the correct patient was killed on a subsequent occasion. In another incident, a family was told someone was dead, but they had not been sent to the killing centres: this error was soon dealt with by simply killing the person anyway.[17]

Protestors

Many families became suspicious as a result of these bureaucratic errors, or simply the sudden death of their relative. Although families in the same district were not meant to receive identical letters, there were nevertheless examples of several different disabled relatives dying at the same time, of the same causes, which created scepticism among the recipients of the notifications. As a result there was some unrest in various local communities, for example Absberg, Bruckberg and Württemberg.

People in the vicinity of the killing centres had also become aware of the activities, due to the smoke and the smell, and the regular arrival of buses that departed without their passengers. For example, a prominent local woman in the vicinity of the Grafeneck centre, Else von Löwis, wrote a protest letter to the wife of Judge Walter Buch in November 1940, which was forwarded to Himmler. Subsequently, Himmler advised Brack, the T-4 director, to close Grafeneck:

> As I have heard, there is great excitement in the Swabian Jura due to the institution Grafeneck. The populace recognises the grey automobiles of the SS, and thinks it knows what is happening under the constant smoke of the crematorium. What takes place there is a secret, and yet it is no longer a secret. Thus the worst public mood has taken hold there, and in my opinion there remains only one option: discontinue the operation of the institution in this locality.[18]

In retrospect, protest at the T-4 programme was almost inevitable. It was impossible to hide the sudden deaths of tens of thousands of people, or to conceal the killing institutions or transports. The T-4 front organizations did not deceive the public, and the regular Nazi propaganda against 'useless eaters' suggested who was behind the disappearances. Unlike the Jewish and Gypsy populations, disabled people were connected to ordinary German families: they were isolated, stigmatized and victimized, but not a separate ethnic enclave.

The legal concern about the euthanasia programme has been noted, as has the resistance of some doctors. But it is worth registering here, as Hugh

Gallagher points out, that of all the letters of protest, only one was written by a psychiatrist. Another salient fact is that Church opposition was very muted and very late, despite the fact that the Protestant Inner Mission organization ran many residential institutions, as did the various Catholic religious orders. They cannot have been unaware of what was happening to their patients after they were driven away in the grey buses.

Gallagher and Friedlander both show that the Protestant Church had not been concerned about the previous development of eugenic sterilization. Protestant theologians involved in the Inner Mission's Standing Conference on Eugenics meeting in 1931 had supported various eugenic principles, and the Protestant Church went on to accept both voluntary and later compulsory sterilization, and indeed to help implement such schemes in its homes. Dr Rudolf Boeckh, the medical director of the Protestant Neuendettelsau asylum in Franconia, had told a local Nazi Party meeting that his residents were 'a travesty of humankind' who deserved to be 're-turned to the Creator': 1,911 of the 2,137 patients were later taken away and murdered.

The Catholic Church was more opposed to sterilization. However, protest was muted because of the Concordat that the Nazis had signed with the Vatican. Catholic bishops made Jesuitical distinctions between passively doing one's duty and actively soliciting another's harm, in order to exonerate Catholic doctors and nurses. When the euthanasia programme started, the Catholic Church tried to secure opt-outs for its own institutions, and negotiated to enable victims to be given the last sacraments.

On realizing that a covert programme of killing was being implemented – with the collection and disappearance of many residents of religious homes – institutions run by both churches initiated various resistance strategies. Some asylums tried to hide vulnerable individuals or ask families to take them home (often without success), or to plea-bargain about particular cases, or to attempt subversion by bureaucratic means. However, success was very limited.

Other clergy were braver and more outspoken. For example, Gallagher describes how in 1940 Pastor Paul Gerhard Braune prepared a report documenting the large-scale operation to eliminate 'unworthy lives', which he took to Kerrl, the Church Affairs Minister, and to Gürtner at the Ministry of Justice. The report was subsequently forwarded to Hermann Goering: Braune was arrested by the Gestapo, interrogated and imprisoned, and he was only released after he had promised not to take further action. Another very prominent Protestant critic was Pastor Friedrich von Bodelschwingh, director of the Bethel Mission. He refused to co-operate in the T-4 programme and protested against the illegal and irreligious policy, asking for it to be stopped and, at the very least, for Bethel to be exempted. He even had long discussions with Brandt. The Nazis did not dare arrest Bodelschwingh and consequently left the Bethel Mission alone: no one from the institution was taken directly to the killing centres.

The most famous Catholic protestor was Clemens August Graft von Galen, Bishop of Munster. He was a conservative and a patriot, but had been very alienated by Nazi attacks on church property. Michael Burleigh notes that he had been informed about the euthanasia programme by Dr Karsten Jaspersen in July 1940. Eventually, he delivered three public sermons against the Nazis in July and August 1941, which were widely reproduced and distributed. The third sermon was an unequivocal condemnation of the T-4 programme as a violation of the Fifth Commandment, in which the bishop stated 'there are obligations of conscience from which no one can release us and which we must discharge even at the cost of our lives'.[19] Bishop Galen also distributed a pastoral letter against euthanasia throughout his diocese, sent protest telegrams to government and army leaders, and sent an official letter reporting the crimes to the district attorney of Münster, asking for the lives of institutionalized patients to be protected. Within a month, both attacks on church property and the T-4 programme ended.

Although the T-4 programme was halted, it should not be assumed that this demonstrates the success of religious protest specifically, as Friedlander shows. First, widespread public opposition had developed, particularly from relatives of murdered patients, and from communities neighbouring the killing centres. Second, by August 1941, the T-4 target of 70,000 victims had already been attained. Third, children's euthanasia, euthanasia in the camps and 'wild' or unofficial euthanasia continued after the order to stop. Finally, T-4 personnel went on to be centrally involved in implementing the extermination of the Jews, and this new priority may have been a factor in the halt of T-4. Friedlander suggests that

> The killers, who had assumed that the program would be welcomed by the majority of the population, were surprised by the strength of public opposition. At first, they believed that they needed only better communications and thus launched a propaganda drive to make the killings acceptable. But propaganda, even the popular entertainment film sponsored by T-4, could not replace legal security, and the regime had to retreat.[20]

Many Germans were disgusted at what was going on, regarding it as both criminal and immoral. Most disabled people had a family network who were concerned about them. There was public opposition to euthanasia, whereas there was less resistance to the subsequent Holocaust because Jewish families were segregated from the mass of ordinary Germans: only where Jewish people were married to Germans was there opposition, and in many of these cases the Jewish spouse escaped deportation and death in the camps.

Conclusion

Although approximately 70,000 people were killed in the official T-4 programme, many more died subsequently: Dr Leo Alexander provided a study of euthanasia for the Nuremberg trials after the war, and he estimated that a total of 275,000 were killed. The number may have been even greater. To take one example, in 1939 there were 300,000 mental patients in Germany; in 1946, there were only 40,000. No wonder that psychiatrists towards the end of the war were becoming worried that they would not have any role to perform in future.

Given this death toll, and the decimation of the disabled population, it is surprising that there is widespread ignorance today of Nazi eugenics and euthanasia. Friedlander argues:

> At the time, the murder of the handicapped led to public opposition, while the murder of Jews, and even more so Gypsies, failed to produce public opposition. Since the war, however, public interest has focussed on the murder of Jews, while the murder of the handicapped and Gypsies has received little attention until recently.[21]

No compensation has ever been given to those sterilized, or to the heirs of those disabled people who were killed.

The enormous evil of the genocidal policy towards the Jewish people of Europe has perhaps overshadowed the equally tragic fate of disabled people in Germany and central Europe. Yet the notions of racial science that lay behind the killings of disabled people led to the subsequent killings of Jews and Gypsies: the same logic, but also the same technology was applied. The history of Nazi racial policy shows the operation of the 'slippery slope', as eugenics became euthanasia, which became the Holocaust. Each stage made the subsequent development more acceptable and more effective, and the perpetrators became more hardened and more willing to perform murderous acts.

A key point to register about Nazi euthanasia is the central involvement of scientists and doctors. It is impossible to write off what happened as the aberrant behaviour of a group of thugs, fanatics and ideologues. It was doctors, not SS men, who killed in the euthanasia centres or on the children's wards. Prejudice against disabled people, and racial minorities, was enshrined in the scientific orthodoxy of the early twentieth century, and most of those involved in sterilizing and killing disabled people felt that they were performing a service both to society and even to the individuals themselves. At post-war trials, many doctors and managers were able to justify their behaviour to themselves, and some refused to accept that they had committed crimes. As Burleigh argues, 'We are dealing with a group of people who believed in the rectitude of what they did, even if they did not care to share their reasoning with the confused traditionalist mass of humanity through some form of explicit legal sanctioning.'[22]

After the war, the German medical profession closed ranks and refused to acknowledge what had happened, or the culpability of many of its members. Some perpetrators were brought to trial, but many escaped justice. For example, many nurses were acquitted, on the defence that they had just followed the orders of physicians. Dr Alexander Mitscherlich, a junior physician, produced a book on the Nuremberg Doctors' Trial that summarized the whole proceedings. Ten thousand copies were printed in 1949 and sent to the West German Physicians' Chambers for distribution. Hugh Gallagher states that the books totally disappeared and were never circulated.

Doctors such as Klaus Enruweit, Hermann Voss, Werner Catel, Julius Hallervorden, Werner Villinger and Werner Heyde all took part in the euthanasia programme and continued practising afterwards. Some changed their names – for example, Werner Heyde became Dr Sawade. Dr Werner Catel, who had been head of the medical committee for children's euthanasia, subsequently became professor of paediatrics and director of the children's clinic at the University of Kiel, although he was later forced to retire. In 1962 he published a book, *Borderline Situations of Life*, setting forth the case for euthanasia of disabled children.

Acknowledgement of medical crimes finally arrived in 1989: a speech was delivered at the German Federal Chamber of Physicians about the moral guilt of the medical profession in Nazi Germany. Only in recent decades has the collection of medical specimens gathered in the euthanasia programme, such as the brains at the Max Planck Institute, been given proper burial and recognition.

4
Eugenics in democratic societies

During 1997, the UK experienced a retrospective media panic about the Swedish eugenic sterilization programme. A period of European history that had been well known among social policy scholars, and extensively discussed in Sweden and other Scandinavian countries, suddenly became of great public interest. Professor Hilary Rose reflects on how this old story became contemporary 'news', and suggests:

> What has happened is that liberal democratic countries, particularly where there has been a strong welfare state, have developed a culture of denial. Our eugenic histories in their unpleasant variety are forgotten; instead the practice of eugenics is solely put at the Nazi door. Demonizing the Nazi demons is fair enough, but not if it enables us to deny our pasts. Both the left and liberal democrats want to forget that an enthusiasm for eugenics was widely spread among the intellectuals of the first half of this century, whether they were geneticists or social policy analysts, social reformers, feminists or marxist revolutionaries.[1]

In this chapter, we consider Scandinavian eugenics, drawing on the work of Bent Sigurd Hansen, Gunnar Broberg and Mattias Tydén, Nils Roll-Hansen and Marjatta Hietala, published together in *Eugenics and the Welfare State: Sterilization policy in Denmark, Sweden, Norway and Finland*. We discuss how eugenic policies were instituted in these liberal democratic societies, and how they continued up to the 1970s, and in some cases beyond.

In the 1920s, the British Eugenic Society conducted an international survey of sterilization, which revealed that the Nordic countries, the USA and Switzerland led the world. The story of eugenics in the European democracies demonstrates how a combination of a belief in progress – particularly scientific progress – together with the primacy of collective and social objectives over individual rights, can contribute to reproductive discrimination against 'inferior' or 'disabled' members of the population.

Denmark (1929), Norway (1934), Sweden (1935) and Finland (1935) each passed and implemented eugenic legislation during the middle

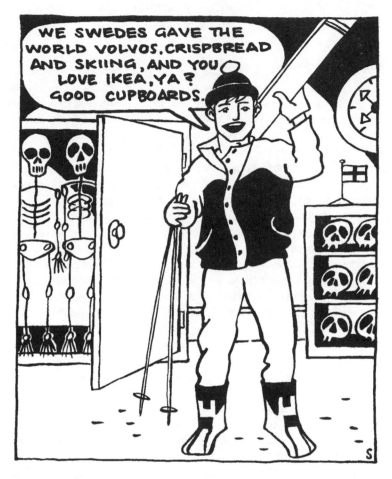

decades of the twentieth century. While each has distinctive features, these countries shared several common elements: all were ethnically rather homogenous, despite some immigration and a significant Sami minority in Finland; the notion of a 'Nordic ideal' was significant; the established Lutheran Church played an important role in society; modernization occurred rapidly in the first decades of the twentieth century, with science and technology playing a vital role in changing society and economy; and finally, in contrast to the rest of Europe, social democratic parties dominated government from the 1920s and 1930s onwards. These social democratic administrations developed strong welfare states, following the example of Sweden which implemented P. A. Hansson's concept of a 'people's home' from 1928. With the exception of the Nazi occupation of Norway and Denmark, the history of these countries is marked by stability, security and consensus.

The path to eugenics

Changes in attitudes to people with learning difficulties played an important part in the development of eugenic practices in these countries. By the end of the nineteenth century, the hope that modern forms of education and cure would reduce the impact of learning difficulties was proving ill-founded. Institutions were becoming places of isolation, limited training and socially useful work, rather than centres of therapy and rehabilitation. Broader changes in society, such as increasing urbanization and industrialization, made people with learning difficulties more visible. While in traditional societies based on family and community disabled people were more integrated, the modern society led to the 'separating out' of those who could not work or live independently, which increased the pressure on institutions and made it appear that people with learning difficulties were a growing problem. These concerns became focused on the 'sexual promiscuity' and 'irresponsibility' that were associated with people with learning difficulties. At the same time, philanthropists were giving way to medical practitioners as leaders of institutions, and the classification and assessment of mental retardation was increasingly emphasized. Often, institutions were run by a family and leadership was passed down through the generations, for example in the case of the Danish Keller family. No wonder there was strong support for hereditarian ideas.

In 1912, the subject of eugenics was raised at the Sixth Nordic Conference on the Welfare of the Handicapped in Helsinki: while many participants opposed the idea, advocates were to continue promoting sterilization and similar policies at successive conferences. Institutions later became the places where eugenic sterilizations were first performed. Medical staff provided observations and data to support eugenic measures, performed the operations and evaluated the benefits. In some cases, sterilization was perceived as an alternative to institutionalization: if segregation arose out of a fear of increasing numbers of people with learning difficulties, sterilization offered the chance to integrate such people back into society, without fear of them reproducing. In Denmark, Hansen tells how Christian Keller had gone to the extent of taking over whole islands – one for men with learning difficulties in 1910, another for women with learning difficulties in 1920. In the same year Keller, on behalf of all institutions for mentally retarded people, asked the government to set up an expert commission to discuss sterilization.

Population concerns

In Finland, Norway and particularly Sweden, anxieties about the population lay behind the support for eugenics. Broberg and Tydén note that at the beginning of the century, one-sixth of the Swedish population emigrated, primarily to the USA. Rapid social change and high social mobility brought insecurity. This was expressed in concern about racial degeneration and immigration, although in 1907, for example, there was a total of only 1,678 foreign workers in Sweden. The racial focus originated in the nineteenth-century tradition, with anthropologists such as Anders Retzius promoting superior Nordic virtues, while Victor Rydberg wrote about the potential downfall of the white race and the threat of the Chinese. There was also interest in the Lapp/Sami people, supposedly an inferior stock to the Swedes.

In 1909 the Swedish Society for Racial Hygiene was formed in Stockholm: it remained small, but influential in medical circles. The physician Herman Lundborg began preaching eugenics as salvation of the nation, stressing the importance of heredity and the danger of degeneration. Broberg and Tydén quote his comment that

> a host of more or less poorly equipped individuals come into being, and they will soon make their will known, especially in periods of unrest or unemployment... We must pay attention to the genotype to a far greater extent than hitherto; that is, we must work far more than is being done now for the lineage and the race, for good families and healthy children.[2]

Lundborg went on to lead the first government Institute for Racial Biology in the world, founded in Uppsala in 1922. This development reflected both the spread of nationalist sentiment after the war – with the failure of social democrat internationalism – as well as the idea of science as the agent for moral improvement and the transformation of society. The Institute's first publication was a statistical volume on *The Racial Character of the Swedish Nation*.

Broberg and Tydén demonstrate that, in Sweden, there was considerable interest and support for German racial ideas in the inter-war period. There was also hostility to Sami, Gypsies and immigrants, despite their low numbers. When Jewish doctors emigrated from Germany to Sweden in 1939, there were student protests in Uppsala, Lund and Stockholm. As well as such xenophobic sentiment, there was growing anxiety about the population in the 1930s, with the falling birth rate: Sweden had the lowest birth rate in the world in 1934. With the change from mainstream to reform eugenics in this period came a concern with the quantity rather than the quality of births, in the work of people like Gunnar Myrdal. Old theories about miscegenation were replaced by genetic searches for hereditary diseases. Yet there was anxiety that social reform, designed to promote the birth rate, might facilitate reproduction among less desirable parents. Thus, Alva Myrdal argued in 1941 that 'the fact that community aid is accompanied by increased fertility in some groups hereditarily defective or in other respects deficient and also the fact that infant mortality among the deficient is decreasing demands some corresponding corrective'.[3] In Norway too, concerns about the population were influential in the move to eugenics, with a halt to population growth and an apparent rise in the number of people with learning difficulties.

In Finland, Hielta notes that eugenic ideas were promoted by the Swedish-speaking minority, who made up an eighth of the population at the turn of the century and dominated the country's elite: racial hygiene was part of a campaign to bolster the position of the Swedish population. It was argued that the Finnish race was inferior to the more Nordic Swedes. Professor Harry Federley led Samfundet, the Swedish-speaking public health organization, which promoted eugenic ideas among Swedish families from 1921. Awards were given to healthy Swedish-speaking mothers who had four or more children: over an eight-year period, 601 mothers received special diplomas, while 211 mothers were given a monetary reward.

However, there was also a strong current of Finnish nationalism. Beauty contests were organized in 1919 and 1926 to improve the image of the Finnish race. There was celebration of the success of Finnish athletes in winning nine gold medals at the Stockholm Olympics of 1912, and there was a major triumph in 1934 when Ester Toivonen was declared Europe's most beautiful woman.

Ideas and advocates

International links played an important role in the spread of eugenic ideas. Often it was attendance at an international eugenics congress that enthused individuals to come home and promote eugenic thinking. Roll-Hansen tells of pharmacist Jon Alfred Mjöen, a key propagandist for race hygiene. He had studied in Germany, later participated in the First International Congress of Eugenics in London in 1912 and joined the Permanent International Committee for Eugenics (chaired by Leonard Darwin), and published a book on race hygiene in 1914. In Denmark, physical anthropologist Søren Hansen also attended the First International Congress of Eugenics, and was converted to enthusiastic advocacy. Bent Sigurd Hansen describes him as 'almost a one-man eugenics movement',[4] lecturing and writing about eugenics in specialist and mainstream publications, and calling for anthropological and genetic research. Hielta notes that Professor Harry Federley of Finland was a delegate to the Third Congress of Eugenics, returning to promote eugenics: he corresponded extensively with Scandinavian and American eugenicists, particularly about concerns over alcoholism and criminality.

In Norway, as in other Scandinavian countries, Roll-Hansen notes that advocates of eugenics tended to be divided between those concerned with racial hygiene and those whose work focused on more mainstream medical concerns. Thus there was a split between Mjöen and his Consultative Eugenics Committee of Norway and the Norwegian Genetics Society, which included reputable physicians such as Otto Mohr, Professor Ragnar Vogt (founder of Norwegian psychiatry) and Kristine Bonnevie (specialist in cytology and genetics). Bonnevie, the first female professor in Norway, set up the Institute of Genetics at the University of Kristiania (Oslo), which researched population groups in the remote Norwegian valleys. She resisted Charles Davenport's 1927 invitation to join the Commission of the International Federation of Eugenic Organizations, favouring research rather than rhetoric. But she remained a prudent and modest supporter of eugenic ideas. Otto Mohr worked at Columbia with Thomas Hunt Morgan on chromosome research, and with increasing knowledge became more critical of eugenics: his popular book of 1923 discussed the importance of environmental factors, and rejected both positive and negative eugenic policies.

For many Scandinavians, it was the influence of the USA, rather than Germany, which led to eugenics. For example, Hansen tells how in 1910 Bodil Hjort, a young woman doctor at the big Keller institution at Bregninge, was funded to visit some of the more famous American institutions, and met Henry H. Goddard, the hereditarian author. This was one of the ways in which Goddard's ideas influenced Danish thinking. In Sweden, Lundborg collaborated with Charles Davenport, of Cold Spring Harbour, on racial research. Later, Christian Keller translated a lecture by Walter Fernald, superintendent of the Massachusetts School for the Feeble-Minded, which promoted a hereditarian ideology, and a eugenic solution.

Many experts on genetics supported the idea of negative eugenics. Hansen notes that in Denmark this included Wilhelm Johannsen, a key supporter of Mendelianism who had coined the terms 'gene', 'genotype' and 'phenotype'. His 1917 monograph on heredity seemed to oppose 'human stockbreeding', promoted the importance of environmental factors and challenged the concept of 'normality', and he argued against the 'haphazard' approach of Americans such as Davenport. Yet he joined the International Eugenics Commission in 1923, and joined the Danish commission on castration and sterilization in 1924, following the marriage law of 1922. During the 1920s he was cautiously supportive of negative eugenics. Other leading geneticists were also supporters of negative eugenics, including the pathologist Oluf Thomsen and the psychiatrist August Wimmer, both convinced hereditarians, and later the mycologist Øivind Winge.

Scandinavian eugenics programmes

Denmark

Bent Sigurd Hansen's study of Danish eugenics tells how the Scandinavian social democrat ideal stressed harmony between classes, the importance of the family and the good of society as a whole. For social reformers such as the Danish social democrat K. K. Steincke, eugenics was a key part of the blueprint of the rational welfare state, as he argued in his 1920 book, *Social Relief of the Future*. His plans combined negative eugenics with a complementary support for social relief. Hansen characterizes his views thus:

> Just to abandon the unfit and helpless would be callous; allowing them to breed unhindered would be folly – but eugenics solved the problem. You could afford to be humane and generous toward them, feed them and clothe them, as long as eugenic measures ensured that they did not increase in number.[5]

We note that this position seems similar to the policy of the modern People's Republic of China. Yet Steincke was also a puritanical elitist, who disapproved of the ignorant masses and the corrupting media. He was revolted by the 'bestial' sexual activity of mentally retarded people in institutions. He felt that the responsible and humanitarian solution was to commission the experts to introduce eugenics.

Steincke's book coincided with the request from Keller on behalf of the Danish institutions, and a 100,000-name petition from the Women's National Council, which was worried about the rise in sexual offences and demanded castration as a solution. Simultaneously, a 1923 law stated that mentally impaired and mentally ill people would henceforth require permission from the minister of justice in order to marry.

Hansen tells how the 1924 social democrat government of Denmark, with Steincke as Secretary of Justice, instituted a commission on sterilization and castration, comprising Wilhelm Johannsen, August Wimmer, Christian Keller and five other representatives of institutions. Its 1926 report, *Social Measures Toward Degeneratively Predisposed Individuals*, surveyed the evidence and statistics on heritability. The commission concluded that legislation directed towards racial improvement was not feasible because sterilization would not reduce the incidence of hereditary conditions. But the commission also argued that it should nevertheless be legitimate to sterilize certain groups, including mentally ill people, who would not be capable of raising children and whose children might also be genetically harmed. Hansen notes that this approach meant that it was not necessary to prove that a particular case was inherited. Sterilization would be limited to people confined to institutions. While this was the most confined group, it was less controversial to sterilize residents of institutions and could also lead to release into the community and consequent relaxation of space pressures on institutions. The second half of the proposal suggested castration for repeat sex offenders. No distinction was made between violent sex offences and sexual behaviours such as exhibitionism and homosexuality, and after the introduction of the law there were some sterilizations of people in the latter category.

It was proposed that there should be a trial period of implementation of the policy, with a complicated procedure by which the Secretary of Justice had to approve recommendations coming from a medical–legal council. There were no clear guidelines on categories or severity of conditions. However, Hansen stresses that the policy was voluntary: consent was needed from anyone who was capable of understanding the operation, or the guardians of those who were not competent to consent in their own right. He also notes that it would have been difficult for people to resist the pressures towards sterilization, and consent was a token process in many cases.

The Sterilization Act was finally approved in 1929, by the new Agrarian Party government, showing the bipartisan consensus that existed on the issue of eugenics. Subsequently, Steincke and the Social Democrats introduced a Mental Handicap Act in 1934, which included measures for compulsory confinement of certain groups of people with learning difficulties. It was to be the duty of teachers, doctors and social authorities to report suspected cases of mental disability. There were two conditions for sterilization: if people were judged unable to raise children, or if the operation would enable them to be released from confinement. The 1934 law extended sterilization to minors and to people outside institutions, did not require the consent of the subject and made the whole procedure more straightforward. Hansen argues that although it did not mention eugenics, this was the first compulsory and universal sterilization measure, under which far more people were sterilized than under the 1929 Act. In 1935, there was a further revision to the 1929 Act, clarifying some of the confusion and narrowing the criteria. Until 1945, 78 per cent of those sterilized were mentally retarded, and of these about twice as many were women as men.

Hansen also tells how, during the 1930s in Denmark, there was hardening of support for the eugenics law. For example, while German racial laws were condemned, the Nazi eugenics policy was warmly welcomed. Søren Hansen called the German law of 1933 'as good as expected'. August Wimmer called for Denmark to adopt the new German practice of compulsory sterilization of psychopaths, alcoholics and criminals. The differences between the two countries' legislation were fairly minor. Although many more people were sterilized in Germany in this period, none of the Danish eugenicists was critical of the extent of the German programme.

Hansen notes that when the medical–legal council reviewed the Danish sterilization experiment in 1935, there was a consensus among medical experts that it was successful and desirable: there were suggestions that it would be beneficial to extend the measures to hereditary blindness and deafness, and even to psychopaths, alcoholics and habitual criminals. When the review was published in the Danish Medical Association periodical, there was no adverse reaction from the profession.

Table 4.1 Sterilizations in Denmark, 1929–50[6]

Period	Women with learning difficulties	Men with learning difficulties	Women without learning difficulties	Men without learning difficulties	Total
1929–34	84	19	4	1	108
1935–39	825	375	150	30	1,380
1940–45	1,000	500	510	110	2,120
1946–50	869	465	902	96	2,332
Total	2,778	1,359	1,566	237	5,940

Norway

Nils Roll-Hansen's study of Norwegian eugenics begins with the proposal of Dr Jon Alfred Mjöen's Consultative Eugenics Committee to the Ministry of Justice in 1931, advocating compulsory segregation and voluntary sterilization to prevent the procreation of people with learning difficulties, as a precaution to avoid the serious danger of racial degeneration. The following year, the penal code revisers published a proposal for a sterilization law, including optional castration for sex offenders. Sterilization was to occur only with the consent of the subject or their guardian, and was to be permitted only for eugenic and social reasons, not for the purpose of contraception.

The Sterilization Law of 1934 allowed sterilization when a person could not take care of children, or if there was a likelihood of passing on hereditary disease; where there was a chance of cure, insane people were not to be sterilized. The law was proposed by Erling Björnsen, a nationalist member of the Farmers' Party who was later to join the Norwegian Nazi Party. Roll-Hansen tells how in his speech he compared population policy to the farmer's management of livestock, said he would have preferred more radical, compulsory law, and expressed gratitude to Mjöen and his committee. But he also notes that other eugenic campaigners in Norway had in fact proposed more coercive policies, in line with the German law of 1933.

As in other Nordic countries, the majority of sterilizations in Norway were of people with learning difficulties, and between 80 and 90 per cent were women. The German Nazis occupied Norway from 1940 to the end of the war. This led to a further extension of the Norwegian programme, starting in 1942, and a sharp increase in sterilization. Roll-Hansen tells how this was marked by a stress on the role of biological inheritance rather than environmental factors, and a subordination of individual rights to the interests of society as a whole. In practical terms, the family or guardian of a person with learning difficulties was no longer allowed to exercise a veto over sterilization, and the use of force was permitted. A new Institute for Biological Heredity was formed at the University of Oslo, headed by Thordar Quelprud. These measures led to a sharp increase in the rate of sterilizations. The average number of sterilizations prior to Nazi takeover was a little below 100 each year. During the two and a half years of Nazi rule, average annual sterilizations numbered around 280. Roll-Hansen notes that throughout this period, the Norwegian genetics establishment co-operated with Nazi population policy.

Finland

Marjatta Hietala tells how in Finland, the government first appointed a committee to investigate a eugenic law in 1926. This group gathered information on legislation in other countries, and statistics on people with learning difficulties; it also canvassed opinion from leaders of institutions, most of whom were in favour of voluntary sterilization measures. The committee's 1929 proposal supported a eugenic law, dependent on the consent of the subject, or guardian if the subject was not legally competent. Scope would be restricted to people with learning difficulties, mental illness or epilepsy, and hereditary deafness: criminality, alcoholism and other anti-social behaviours were not permitted justifications. As Hietala comments, the use of sensationalist vignettes in the report added rhetorical weight to the arguments for sterilization.

During the 1930s, the impact of economic depression meant that increasing numbers of poor families were dependent on state support, which fuelled debates on eugenic measures: nearly 10 per cent of the population were receiving welfare relief. Hietala identifies concern about criminality as another element in the growing demand for eugenic legislation – Harry Federley and others were arguing that criminality depended on genotype, not circumstances, often referencing German sources. She also notes that women on both sides of the political divide supported sterilization of sex offenders and child abusers. These various factors meant that the Sterilization Bill of 1934 had an easy passage through Parliament, coming into force in 1935.

The Act allowed for compulsory sterilization of 'idiots, imbeciles and the insane', in cases where the impairment was believed to be heritable, or where the subject could not care for children. Voluntary sterilization was permitted if it was feared that people would produce inferior children. Sterilization was also allowed for those guilty of actual or attempted crime, 'demonstrating an unnatural sexual drive either in terms of its strength or direction'. Applications for sterilization were to be made in writing to the National Board of Health.

Later, further legislation was introduced to extend the policy, which many felt was not having enough impact. Hietala notes that in the post-war period, there were feelings of rootlessness and anxiety about sexual and violent crime in Finland. The 1950 Sterilization Act allowed operations on eugenic, social or general medical grounds. A consultant and a surgeon were allowed to decide in cases of medical grounds, leading to an increase in such procedures, often in combination with abortion. Hietala notes that 1958 saw eugenic motivations peak, accounting for 19 per cent of all sterilizations (413 sterilizations). The 1950 Castration Act allowed the procedure on the basis of criminal policy and on humanitarian grounds in cases of attempted or actual sexual crime, and where institutionalized people were sexual dangers. There was strong opposition to this measure, which was introduced just as the death penalty was abolished. Because of this controversy, castration was hardly ever applied. From 1951 to 1968, there were 2,777 applications for sterilizations, but only 90 cases went ahead.

Hietala's analysis of the statistics on Finnish sterilization shows that the majority of operations were directed by the authorities, not requested by the patient. A higher proportion of Finnish speakers than Swedish speakers were sterilized. Often, poorer local authorities resorted to sterilization because they felt they could not afford to maintain people with learning difficulties out of public funds. After the 1950s, eugenic sterilization declined, as a higher proportion of operations were carried out to enable women to limit their families.

As Hietala argues, the eugenics programmes in Finland were linked to perceptions that the population was declining in quantity as well as quality: this was a particular fear of the dominant Swedish-speaking minority. Medicine was regarded with great respect, as a modernizing force: expertise was admired, and the majority of Finnish doctors supported eugenic sterilization. Eugenics was another example of the Finnish adoption of foreign practices, rather than being a home-grown idea.[7]

Sweden

Broberg and Tydén's study of Swedish eugenics tells how a Sterilization Bill was introduced in 1922 by psychiatrist Alfred Petrén, with some cross-party support. The bill emphasized the economic benefits of avoiding the burden of institutional care of mentally retarded and mentally ill people, and the social danger of unfit parenting. Following this initiative, and calls for eugenic measures from the Institute for Race Biology in 1923 and from the National Board of Health in 1924, a commission was set up to discuss the issue in 1927, comprising four experts (two medical, one lawyer, one psychiatrist). Their 1929 report proposed a very restrictive law, limited to voluntary sterilization on genetic grounds of hereditary disease, but not social grounds. The report was widely criticized. However, sterilizations continued to be performed on eugenic grounds throughout the 1920s, despite their illegality.

Broberg and Tydén note that in 1933, after Petrén had revived the issue of a sterilization law, the Swedish Parliament asked Ragnar Bergendal, a Professor of Criminal Law, to investigate its potential. His report proposed sterilization of legally incompetent individuals without the need for consent and despite any parental opposition: he argued that the interests of society should outweigh those of individuals, and that, perhaps, it was even better not to inform patients of the nature of the operation. In 1934, the Social Democrat government put forward a Sterilization Bill along these lines, which became law at the beginning of the following year. Sterilization without consent was to be permitted in the case of mental illness, feeble-mindedness or other mental defects, in cases where the patient was legally incompetent or incapable of caring for children, or if they were likely to transmit mental illness or feeble-mindedness. It was necessary to apply to the National Board of Health for permission, except in cases of mental retardation where two physicians could decide jointly.

Broberg and Tydén discuss how, during the 1930s, the debate on eugenics widened. The focus spread beyond mental deficiency to 'socially maladjusted' individuals – prostitutes, vagrants and people considered to be workshy. There was no questioning of the value or acceptability of sterilization. In the discussions leading to the stronger eugenics legislation of 1941, the need to purify the Swedish racial stock was a strong theme. For example, Social Democrat Karl Johan Olsson said in Parliament: 'I think it is better to go a little too far than to risk bringing unfit and inferior offspring into the world.' Others called for the compulsory sterilization of all anti-social elements and for coercive enforcement of eugenic principles. The 1941 Sterilization Act extended the 'eugenic grounds' to persons suffering from severe physical diseases or defects of a hereditary nature, as well as mental retardation or mental illness. 'Social grounds' were expanded to include anti-social lifestyles as well as mental retardation and mental illness. The Act also allowed for the voluntary sterilization of women for medical reasons.

The Swedish eugenics legislation reflected the same motives as the contemporary German laws, although it was applied in a more limited and less coercive fashion, relying on persuasion, not force. However, Broberg and Tydén note that many mentally retarded girls were sterilized before leaving special schools or homes. Sometimes sterilization was a condition for discharge. Subsequent sterilization was also sometimes a condition for abortion to be carried out for certain categories of women. The majority of sterilization procedures were carried out on women, despite the fact that the operation was simpler to perform on males, which arguably reflects the lower status of women in Swedish society at the time. While the eugenics policy was cloaked in scientific language, case reports include much personal opinion and prejudice, with issues of morals and lifestyle taken into account when deciding on sterilization. Social problems such as vagrancy and alcoholism were often discussed in racial terms, and travellers ('Tattare') and others on the fringes of Swedish society were seen as a threat.

While Sweden introduced its eugenic law at the same time as other Scandinavian countries, it proved far more efficient in implementing eugenics. Broberg and Tydén document the sterilization of 3,000 people under the first law, and a total of 63,000 under both laws (1935–75). While eugenic grounds continued as one reason for sterilization up until the 1960s, the majority of sterilizations in these later years were of women who wished to limit the size of their families. The proportion of the population who had been sterilized was 0.9 per 10,000 in 1940; 3.3 per 10,000 in 1950; and 2.2 per 10,000 in 1960. While the eugenic policy had a 'scientific' rationale that was about humane efficiency, the reality was of authoritarian measures and anonymous secret violence.

Opposition to eugenics

It is also important to explore the various currents of opposition to eugenic policies. In Denmark, Hansen notes that this opposition came mainly from the small minority of Catholics. For example, science historian Gustav Scherz argued that knowledge of heredity was incomplete, and that sterilization was a violation of the body created by God. Immorality and promiscuity might increase when fear of pregnancy was removed. The birth rate was already declining, and so reproduction should not be further suppressed. In general, this was an opposition not to eugenic ideas, to conservative notions about racial quality or to hereditarianism, but to the method of sterilization. It was associated with Catholic attacks on social democracy and parliamentarism, which also included an undercurrent of anti-Semitism. The Danish Lutheran Church showed no opposition to sterilization whatsoever, according to Hansen.

The only parliamentary opposition to the Danish law of 1929 came from a small group within the Conservative Party led by clergyman Alfred Bindslev, on the basis that life should not be meddled with in this way, and that little was really known about these issues. Having failed to stop the legislation, this group continued to fight against successive eugenic measures, always in vain. In society at large, teachers resisted eugenic approaches, for example when slow but normal children fell below the IQ minimum level and were removed to institutions. Parents also opposed the transfer of their children. Protest was primarily against forcible confinement, however, rather than against eugenic sterilization. Authorities ascribed such opposition to ignorance, and medical professionals continued to insist on their expertise to decide.

In Finland, Hietala notes that there was parliamentary opposition from some who felt that the eugenics legislation had class motives. Professor of Anatomy Matti Väinö also spoke in opposition, citing many examples of famous men who would never have been born if such an act had been in operation. In Norway, Roll-Hansen notes that the only parliamentary opposition came from the single member of the Social Rights Party, who argued from the rights of the individual and upheld the role of social factors rather than biological ones. The argument about encroachment on personal rights was not a salient feature in the Swedish debate either, according to Broberg and Tydén. The dominant response to concern or opposition was the suggestion that the public needed to be educated to accept the policy.

In the decades after the war, eugenic policies slowly declined across the Nordic countries. Hansen notes that in Denmark, there were no post-war recriminations against eugenics, which nevertheless disappeared as a concept. Ongoing resentment against the 1934 Mentally Handicapped Act, including a court case and inquiry, led to a change in 1954 whereby people could appeal decisions on compulsory institutionalization in the courts. Subsequent reports in 1957 and 1958 recommended that the compulsory element in the 1934 law be rescinded, and criticised compulsory sterilization. Finally, in 1967, compulsory sterilization and castration were removed from the law. However, release from institutions could still depend on previous sterilization, so pressure could still be exerted on people to have the operation. There had been a decline in the number of mentally retarded sterilizations from 275 in 1949 to 80 in 1962, and more safeguards had been put in place. Just as eugenic sterilization was introduced with caution and maybe stealth, so it disappeared quietly from Danish consciousness, according to Hansen. In 1973, free sterilization and abortion were legalized for everybody.

Roll-Hansen notes that in Norway, there was no immediate reduction in sterilization after the end of the war: numbers only declined around 1950. Many still argued in favour of the sterilization of mentally retarded people during this period. The Sterilization Law of 1934 remained in force until 1977, with a minor change in 1961 emphasizing the rights of the individual. While the new law of 1977 placed the initiative firmly on the person to be sterilized, it also permitted voluntary sterilization of people over 25 years without official application, and still permitted involuntary sterilization of individuals if there was a danger of serious illness or deformation, or if they were incapable of caring properly for children.

In Finland, Hietala tells how the eugenics policy was finalled replaced by the 1970 legislation on sterilization, castration and abortion. This law removed compulsory sterilization or castration, and prohibited sterilization for individuals under the age of 18. Permission of a guardian was needed for sterilization of mentally ill or retarded persons. In line with other western nations, the new Abortion Act stressed mental, social and psychological factors, as well as a threat to the life or health of the woman, rather than eugenic indications.

In Sweden, Broberg and Tydén note that in 1956 the Institute for Race Biology changed its name to the Department of Medical Genetics. While old attitudes may have continued, terminology changed: the focus switched from population to families and individuals. By the 1970s, there was strong criticism of compulsory sterilization of people with learning difficulties, and finally, in 1975, all sterilizations without consent were prohibited.

Conclusion

This chapter has focused on the eugenic programmes of Scandinavia. However, it should be noted that other European countries, including France, Austria and Switzerland, also have their own eugenic past, along with other parts of the world including Canada and Japan. For example, Japan passed a National Eugenic Law along German lines in 1940, and another Eugenic Protection Law in 1948. Under the latter legislation, 16,520 people with mental illness or learning difficulties were sterilized between 1949 and 1994, of whom 69 per cent were women. Many disabled women were given hysterectomies against their will in the post-war period.[8]

Most sterilization laws introduced in Europe during the 1930s occurred in countries with Protestant, mainly Lutheran, traditions: the Church may have been uncomfortable with eugenic policies, but it kept quiet about its reservations. Norway, Sweden and Denmark were culturally and socially homogeneous, with strong welfare states and faith in science and progress and efficiency. As Broberg and Tydén comment: 'The ambition to clear away what was old, dirty and diseased could range from a commitment to physical hygiene to an aspiration to create, by means of a eugenic program, a sound and healthy people free from defective genes.'[9] The USA, rather than Germany, was the main model for Scandinavian eugenics. Away from the consensual societies such as those of Scandinavia, countries such as the Netherlands and Great Britain failed to implement eugenics legislation, due to traditions of vigorous parliamentary opposition and independent thinking. But as we shall go on to discuss, a moderate, diffuse form of eugenics continued to flourish in post-war Britain and the USA.

5
Reform eugenics from the 1930s to the 1970s

Much of the international popularity of mainline eugenics began to decline in the 1930s. As Kevles notes, in 1932 the Third International Congress of Eugenics attracted fewer than 100 people. This decline intensified after the war as research put paid to some of the more outlandish claims about heredity, degeneracy and poverty. The horrors of the Nazi Holocaust further undermined the case for population improvement. But it was the changing political and economic context that really undermined the mainline credo. As Mazumdar notes of the British context,

> The eugenic problematic had grown out of the union of a middle-class activism focused upon the pauper class, with a biological view of human failings. In the egalitarian world of welfare and economic growth, the pauper class had disappeared. A class analysis no longer carried weight, and with the loss of the class dimension the eugenic problematic could no longer survive in its original form.[1]

Eugenics reconfigured into a more respectable, medically oriented reform eugenics in the post-war period. This meant that human genetics was then relatively moribund until around the 1950s when geneticists began to make headway with studies of rare and serious disorders, such as the inborn errors of metabolism. But it was not until the 1960s, as chromosomal testing via amniocentesis developed, that the laboratory and the clinic merged once more.

In this chapter we cover the rise of reform eugenics, tracing it through the 1930s up to the early 1970s, when recombinant DNA was developed. We focus on the genetic, medical and scientific knowledge and technology that contributed to reform eugenics, in addition to the practices and rhetoric of the genetics profession and their colleagues in science and medicine more generally. We also consider the social, cultural and political changes in this era, reflecting on how they shaped and reflected developments in genetics and the changing priorities of eugenics. We emphasize the growth of reform eugenics and human genetics *out of* mainline eugenics. Although the word 'eugenics' had been carefully dropped by all but the most extreme by the 1970s, we argue that many of the priorities and much of the rhetoric of eugenics continued in human genetics.

Reforming eugenics

A variety of scientific and cultural trends contributed to the reformation of eugenics in the 1930s and 1940s. Drawing on recent knowledge of blood groups, leading eugenicists like R. A. Fisher began to investigate the linkage between disease and particular blood groups in order to understand their patterns of inheritance. His research unit also maintained an interest in blood and race, at a time when the old notions of biological race were being increasingly criticised in the scientific community. As a result of these studies, Bell and Haldane linked colour blindness and haemophilia in men. Mazumdar shows that this work produced few notable results. Yet this did not hamper the beginnings of human population genetics. Instead these early studies allowed geneticists to hone their statistical and mathematical techniques in the study of large populations and revealed much about the inheritance of blood groups that was of value in its own right.

Around this time Lionel Penrose was also conducting his famous study of the inmates of the Royal Eastern Counties Institution in Colchester. Although he disagreed vociferously with eugenics, he too was motivated by what Mazumdar has called the 'eugenic problematic'; indeed, his study was partly funded by the Eugenics Society in response to the Wood Report on Mental Deficiency in 1929, which identified a large 'social problem group' whose deficiencies were said to be genetically determined. Penrose's research nevertheless undermined the mainline theories of mental and moral deficiency. He revealed the link between what was still called mongolism (now known as Down's syndrome) and maternal age, thus disproving the hereditary thesis. He also undermined what he called a 'facile classification' of mental deficiency, emphasizing instead its multiple causes. He demonstrated a recessive pattern of inheritance to phenylketonuria (PKU) and a dominant pattern to Huntington's disease. In other work with his wife Margaret, they showed that the blood of people with Down's syndrome was not like that of the people of Mongolia, as was previously thought. These findings were an important contribution to the emerging discipline of human genetics, where mental and physical disorders were carefully classified, and their patterns of inheritance were examined using up-to-date mathematical and statistical analysis.

The studies of inheritance in the fruit fly by the Mendelian geneticist T. H. Morgan and colleagues formed yet another plank on which modern genetics was built. Morgan and his team found that genes were positioned on the chromosomes, which determined heredity. His work on evolution and genetics led him to the view that genetic superiority could not be ascribed to whole groups. Thomas resigned from the American Breeders Association during the First World War because of its eugenic sympathies and consistently argued against the association of social deviance with heredity. By the 1930s he had been joined by an increasing number of geneticists.

Attitudes to mental deficiency were also changing in the UK during the 1930s. The war stimulated mental health services (due to the level of psychiatric illness amongst soldiers), which led to a corresponding decline in interest amongst the psychiatric profession in mental defectives. Thomson notes that it also meant that so-called high-grade defectives began to be released from institutions to work in the community. Kevles notes that links between race, class and IQ were also renegotiated in this period, in the USA and the UK. Inspired by Franz Boas, one of the earlier critics of IQ, Otto Klineberg began to study the effects of environment on racial differences in IQ. In the UK, other psychologists' work also ran counter to that of Cyril Burt on intelligence and class, stressing the role of the environment rather than heredity. Kevles notes that, although two important Scottish studies of intelligence in 1932 and 1947 could be interpreted as evidence for the eugenicists' case because they showed that larger families' scores were lower than smaller families', the rise in their mean score was used by critics of eugenics, such as Penrose, to undermine the eugenicists' case for a progressive national decline in intelligence. Watt notes how Penrose also argued that the population's intelligence maintained a natural equilibrium given that 'parents of severe defectives are predominantly of normal or higher intelligence and that a proportion of the offspring of subcultural defectives are of higher intelligence than their parents'.[2] And he argued that it was advantageous for species to be variable (i.e. to possess some bad genes as well as good genes) because changes in the environment (political as well as biological) may mean that bad genes become good, and vice versa.

These criticisms, and others like them, undermined the more extreme elements of the mainline eugenic ideology, while preserving other principles. This is well illustrated in the case of Lionel Penrose. Although a formidable critic of eugenics, all the more so because of his practical and logical deconstruction of the mainline credo, Penrose was still comfortable to extend his expert status beyond the bounds of the laboratory or the clinic to the future of the human race. He shared many of his colleagues' concerns about the population's intelligence and the extent of mental deficiency. Similarly, he was concerned about the quality of the gene pool and engaged in considerable dialogue with C. P. Blacker, the president of the Eugenics Society in Britain, despite his distaste for mainline thinking. As the movement declined, eventually fragmenting into extreme racism on the one hand and obscure learned society on the other, a kind of compromise was reached between scientists and eugenicists, for all their public antagonism. Scientists reworked the old concerns of the past into smaller, more manageable projects focused on disease, and eugenicists tried to bring the new methods of statistical analysis to bear on their traditional interests (in so-called problem families, for example). Although the latter were largely a flop, their legacy continued in the hereditarian wing of psychology, even when it became extremely unfashionable.

In the 1940s medical genetics was in its infancy. Little was known about how to predict, let alone treat, hereditary diseases, save that much of the early eugenic research was simplistic and flawed. The Eugenics Records Office in the USA had been closed and much of its data was dismissed. There were very few clinics devoted to advising people about genetic diseases. One of the first was the Bureau of Human Heredity, opened in London in 1936 (sponsored by the Medical Research Council) to advise on the risks of genetic diseases in affected families. Very few texts existed either. John Fraser Roberts authored *An Introduction to Medical Genetics* in 1940, but physicians and scientists showed little interest in this emerging discipline. Kevles notes that physicians were interested in common diseases like tuberculosis and in diseases that they could treat with new pharmaceuticals like antibiotics. The obscure character of many genetic diseases, and the lack of clear knowledge about patterns of inheritance, diagnostic strategies and treatments, did nothing to increase medical genetics' popularity. Its eugenic associations also played a big part in its unpopularity.

However, eugenics stimulated other interest and support on which human genetics depended. As Paul points out, the majority of the sponsors of human genetics at this time had eugenic motives, including the Rockefeller Foundation. Scientists too were generally supportive of the broad principles of reform eugenics, a term that did not lose its credibility until the 1970s. Part of this new spirit of reform eugenics was an emphasis on environment as well as heredity. For example, the Geneticists' Manifesto, written by Hermann J. Muller and 22 other British and American scientists in 1939, declared that their aim was to achieve the best children possible, whether by heredity or environmental improvements. The development of the 'Modern Synthesis' between the population genetics of

Darwinian theory and classical Mendelian genetics also undercut mainline eugenic ideology. As Kaye points out, 'fitness' was now viewed in terms of reproductive success, not racial superiority, and evolution was thought of as acting on gene frequencies, not individuals.

By the mid-1940s, human genetics was of interest to a small but broad range of specialists from fields as varied as statistics, genetics, psychology, biochemistry and physiology. According to Kevles, the human genetics community of this time numbered around 200. Half the leading members were drawn from physics, and the majority were British. Kevles notes, somewhat wryly, that genetics at this time was not nearly as prestigious as physics and chemistry, although it benefited from the increased funding that these sciences generated. But, as Kaye discusses, the physicists who switched to genetics brought with them a conviction that the mysteries of heredity could be solved and they were keen to overthrow the hypothetical notion of the gene in favour of something more concrete.

Thanks to their efforts, the notion of the gene did begin to take on physical dimensions. Knowledge about the gene's mutation rates and spontaneous mutations developed from earlier blood studies as well as animal and plant genetics in the USA. In 1944 Oswald T. Avery and colleagues suggested that DNA might be the physical substance behind the abstract concept of the gene. Beadle and Tatum at Stanford established the one gene–one enzyme relationship in 1948. Linus Pauling's work on sickle cell haemoglobin and James Neel's identification of its recessive pattern of inheritance, as well as Pauling's development of electrophoresis, a new technique to separate the molecular constituents of substances, were other important developments. As the physical picture of the gene developed, genetic reductionism blossomed.

Genetics became a more significant part of biology in the 1950s. The establishment of the National Health Service in the UK, and the development of treatments for diabetes and anaemia alongside antibiotics, also enhanced the perception of its medical potential. Medical specialists such as paediatricians also became more interested in rare genetic diseases as the more common diseases were successfully treated. Genetic research intensified. In 1953 researchers at the Birmingham Children's Hospital found that variations in diet could mitigate against the effects of PKU. Neel's work on radiation also significantly enhanced the study of populations and consanguinity in human genetics. Meanwhile, knowledge of the chromosomes was also developing. In 1956 Tijo and Levan identified 46 chromosomes (previously thought to be 48) in legally aborted human embryos in Sweden. Around this time women with Turner's syndrome were also found to have only one X chromosome, and an extra chromosome was found in people with Down's syndrome. As the techniques of electrophoresis improved and their costs decreased, they were adopted by a range of laboratories and applied to both normal and 'diseased' populations.

However, eugenics was far from banished to the past. Although Penrose changed the name of the *Annals of Eugenics* to the *Annals of Human Genetics* in 1954, the links between human genetics and eugenics continued, at the institutional and local levels. For example, Paul notes that five out of six presidents of the American Society for Human Genetics were also members of the Eugenics Society's board of directors. She also demonstrates convincingly that the early genetics clinics, although few in number, were often eugenically inspired. These included the Heredity Clinic at the University of Michigan, the Dight Institute at the University of Minnesota and the Genetics Advisory Clinic at the Great Ormond Street Hospital for Sick Children in London, set up by John Fraser Roberts. The patron of the Dight Institute, Charles Fremont Dight, specifically left his estate to the University of Minnesota to promote eugenics. Various important geneticists also applauded the eugenic significance of genetic clinics. Paul cites Gordon Allen, who referred approvingly to 'clinical eugenics', and James Neel, who advocated a 'new eugenics' in 1954.

This was the era of biochemical genetics, bringing together specialists from biochemistry, cytology, anthropology, biophysics, enzymology, embryology and electron microscopy. This network proved particularly productive, focusing on the structure and function of genes and their products. In 1953 Francis Crick and James Watson explained the structure of DNA. In 1955 scientists at the Sanger Laboratory sequenced the amino acids of insulin, firmly establishing that proteins were composed of amino acids. Ingham also found that the haemoglobin in sickle cell disease differed by one amino acid from normal haemoglobin. Jacques Monod and Francis Jacob continued what Kaye has described as this 'conceptual revolution' when they explained the direct role played by DNA in the regulation and co-ordination of the chemical activities in the human body in 1959. Kaye notes that, for Crick, the implication of these new theories was clear: the unity of the genetic code suggested the unity of life and challenged the belief in the uniqueness of humanity. He did much to emphasize the simplicity of DNA, describing it in terms such as the 'code of life' and used it as a battering ram against all that he despised about religion, especially its emphasis on the sanctity of the individual.

Towards molecular genetics

By the end of the 1950s a new molecular biology was beginning to emerge. This was based upon a highly reductionist approach to human biology that extended beyond the bounds of the laboratory to society at large. As Paul argues, Crick and Watson's discovery of DNA 'emboldened' geneticists with eugenic sympathies, as did concerns about the genetic effects of radiation. Crick was amongst the vanguard of this eugenic revival, calling in 1961 for the establishment of a large-scale eugenics programme, which included the sterilization of the citizenry through food additives. Gudding notes how the growing sense of the fragility of both the human body and the body politic also gave succour to the new genetic determinism.[3]

Throughout the 1950s and 1960s, clinical and laboratory-based genetics became increasingly aligned. The importance of medical genetics grew as it was applied in the clinic. Although genetics was still not widely taught in medical schools or colleges, and most researchers in the field were self-taught, the number of genetics clinics had risen to 30 by the late 1960s. These were mostly run by doctors in the UK, and by scientists with PhDs in the USA, but both groups retained eugenic sympathies. Paul notes:

> Throughout the 1960s, most of the leading figures in medical genetics – including Oliver, Curt Stern, Lee R. Dice, Herluf Strandskoz, Gordon Allen, William Allan, C. Nash Heron, Franz Kallmann and Harold Falls, Madge Macklin, and F. Clarke Fraser in the United States and Canada, Eliot Slater and Cedric Carter in Britain and Tage Kemp in Denmark – bluntly described their work as a form of 'eugenics'.[4]

These geneticists sought to distinguish a 'good medical eugenics' from what were characterized as the abuses and bad science of the past. They emphasized rational reproductive decision making. But eugenic sentiments lingered. As Resta has noted, genetic counsellors' emphasis on neutrality 'was a reaction to the methodology of eugenics, not its principles'.[5] Eliminating 'bad' genes that caused diseases like Tay-Sachs or Huntington's was still a priority. Genetic counsellors could at times be quite explicit about their duty to advise their clients, given their responsibility for the population's health. This meant that genetic counselling was far from non-directive.

Treatments for genetic diseases could also be based on eugenic motives. Robert Guthrie's blood test for PKU led to the introduction of newborn screening for the condition in the USA and the UK. Commercially prepared diets also became available as a form of treatment. These were hailed as a great success, partly because they would reduce the costs of treating children with the disease – a public health argument with implicit eugenic connotations. Treatment of PKU was regarded as a form of prevention, similar to genetic counselling to 'control conception', in the words of one commentator.[6]

Even geneticists who did not go so far as to equate human genetics and eugenics acknowledged the importance of eugenics in discussions of human genetics. They frankly discussed eugenic problems such as the ineffectiveness of sterilization and selective breeding, the inability to identify carriers prior to the onset of diseases like Huntington's disease, and the dysgenic effects of treatments.[7]

Geneticists also paved the way for later developments that would dramatically change clinical practice. They discovered that numerous alternative genes could exist at one position (locus) as they sought to identify the primary biochemical deficiencies in genetic diseases. Gudding notes how the responsiveness of genes to their environment was also established, further intensifying genetic determinism.[8] Scientists studied the effects of genes in vitro through new developments such as mouse–human hybrids. DNA was duplicated in a test-tube and a bacterial gene was isolated in the late 1960s. Linkage studies also continued, although these were less successful, focusing as they did on chromosomal rather than genetic abnormalities.

Research into gene therapy also began in the 1960s. Drawing on older concepts of 'biological engineering' articulated by early geneticists such as Haldane and Muller, as well as the Rockefeller Foundation in the 1930s and 1940s, some notable scientists, such as Tatum, Hotchkiss and Szybalski, began to consider genetic modification of humans. As Paul Martin shows, two 'visions' of gene therapy then emerged, based on germ-line and somatic engineering.[9] The first was more classically eugenic and aimed to modify the genetic constitution of future generations, whereas the second was more reformist in its emphasis on treatment of the individual.

These developments prompted considerable public discussion about the possibilities of a 'biological revolution'. As Martin argues, although a positive futuristic discourse was present, considerable anxieties about the creation of a 'super-race' were also expressed, by scientists as well as lay people. But the pronouncements of leading geneticists also retained a decidedly eugenic flavour that echoed the coercive and pessimistic elements of the older mainline eugenics. In 1968 Linus Pauling famously called for compulsory testing of young people for sickle cell anaemia and other deleterious genes, and for them to be tattooed if found to be carriers. Kevles notes that Hermann J. Muller also investigated the possibility of establishing a Foundation for Germinal Choice, where he planned to offer artificial insemination using the sperm of outstanding scientific donors. A foundation was established after his death in 1967, against the wishes of his widow. Although it was greeted with widespread ridicule, Kevles notes that Muller's original proposals were enthusiastically welcomed by many in the scientific and medical communities, including Ernst Mayr, James F. Crow (population geneticist) and Francis Crick, who also toyed with the idea of a licensing scheme to limit the children of the genetically undesirable. Alan Emery also respectfully cited Muller's ideas in his 1968 Inaugural Lecture at the University of Edinburgh.[10]

As genetics became more influential, physicians also became more interested in treating genetic disease. Treatments like the infusion of plasma to replace enzymes lost in certain genetic diseases were attempted, but met with limited success. The possibilities of organ transplant, or 'DNA-mediated transformation of human cells in tissue cultures' were also explored.[11] The treatment of PKU with special diets was also hailed as a great success story of genetic medicine, despite considerable problems with the screening programme, as we will see below.

But it was prenatal diagnosis that really came to the fore in this period. As eugenics became a term of abuse, amniocentesis and the liberalization of abortion presented a radically different genetic service to potential parents. For many this offered the possibility of children where previously they would have elected to remain childless. The ability to detect and abort defective foetuses also allowed a more targeted, individualized, control of human heredity. Amniocentesis was fundamental to this new strategy for eliminating genetic disease. Ruth Schwartz Cowan notes that the amniotic tap had been in use during a pregnant woman's third trimester since the mid-1950s to test for Rh factor disease. In 1955 it was discovered that analysing foetal cells in amniotic fluid could predict the sex of the foetus. As knowledge of the chromosomal abnormalities grew, genetic counselling could now provide information about the genetic make-up of foetal cells. In 1960 a group of doctors in Copenhagen performed an abortion on a male foetus whose mother was a carrier of haemophilia (a disease exclusive to males).[12] The abortion of defective foetuses had begun.

Although sex-linked tests remained relatively rare outside of Scandinavia until the mid-1970s, during the 1960s doctors developed tests for around 100 chromosomal abnormalities in the foetus and screening for Down's syndrome began to be offered to pregnant women over 35 in the UK. Kevles notes that as early as 1961, 131 out of 145 health authorities in England and Wales had introduced such screening tests. Paul notes that the American government also heavily promoted amniocentesis because of its potential to prevent disability and therefore save money. Prenatal diagnosis was also attempted for sickle cell anaemia in the mid-trimester and the possibilities of using knowledge of linkage in prenatal diagnosis was under investigation (and used in one case of myotonic dystrophy).

To facilitate this expansion of genetic testing, genetic counselling began to professionalize. The first master's-level course in genetic counselling in the USA was offered in 1969. Emphasis was placed upon neutral estimations of risk and balanced information, including details of the accuracy of the information provided. Good-quality technical detail was of paramount importance. But the 'deficit model' of patients' understanding still prevailed. Where misunderstandings occurred they were blamed on clients' lack of emotional or mathematical competence, not inadequate or confused information. Impartiality and the client's 'right to decide' were also stressed, reflecting the new attitude to reproduction. As Paul comments: 'within two decades, reproduction was transformed from a public to a private concern'.[13]

But counselling remained skewed in favour of abortion, despite counsellors' rhetoric to the contrary. The culture of intervention and medicalization of disability prevailed as geneticists continued to stress the importance of genetic testing to help parents to 'produce a normal child', in the words of Victor McKusick,[14] or the benefits of 'substantially reducing the emotional and economic burden of many genetic disorders by selective abortion', as Martin and Hoehn put it.[15] Others took a more explicitly eugenic line. For example, Joseph Fletcher argued that no one had the right to knowingly pass on a genetic disease.[16] The dysgenic effects of prenatal diagnosis and treatment in the case of recessive disorders were also a cause for concern.

Various genetic screening programmes were also established in the 1960s and 1970s, under the banner of public health. For example, PKU screening was introduced in 43 states in the USA, beginning in 1963 in Massachusetts. Edelson and Paul have argued that this reflected a convergence of interests amongst clinical geneticists, physicians working in mental institutions, parents and public officials.[17] The screening programmes offered clinical geneticists the opportunity to increase their profile and enabled physicians to ally their work to contemporary medical science. They also offered parents and public officials hope about future treatments. This occurred despite concerns about the accuracy of the test and the knowledge on which it was based.

Paul notes that initially the PKU diet was found to be wanting, as children often still developed learning difficulties, especially if they stopped the diet or if pregnant women did not go on the diet before conceiving and throughout pregnancy. She notes that difficulties posed by the high cost of the diet were not well researched, but undoubtedly also played an important part in the failure of PKU screening and treatment to meet its targets. Notwithstanding these problems, she notes that supporters and detractors of genetics portrayed PKU as a model of a genetic disease that can be treated. For critics of genetics this was useful in underlining the interaction of genes and the environment, to counter what many viewed as the crude genetic determinism of research into genes and IQ. For supporters of genetics, but not necessarily behavioural genetics, PKU was also an illustration of the power of genetics to do good. Paul writes: 'PKU screening was transformed into a simple success story during the 1970s when it became a weapon in the controversy over the genetics of intelligence.'[18]

The prevention of carriers from breeding also stayed on the agenda in this period, although this was now framed in terms of the rights of minority communities to determine their own affairs, rather than the importance of imposing eugenic controls on their reproduction. Tay-Sachs is known to disproportionately affect Ashkenazi Jews, and a register operated by Orthodox Rabbis was established in certain areas of the USA in order to avoid two carriers from marrying and having affected children. In contrast to the success of this scheme, sickle cell screening was more controversial. This was established in the 1970s, partly in response to the growing climate of civil rights activism amongst black Americans (the disease is more prevalent in black people). Ironically, this was to become a source of further discrimination, in contrast to its original aims. In 1972 Congress passed the National Sickle Cell Anemia Control Act and screening laws were in place in several states, some of which made it compulsory. Black people were targeted and employers and legislators alike often confused carrier status with the disease: testing therefore resulted in some overt discrimination, such as the ban on people with sickle cell trait from the air force.

Early screening legislation in the USA was superseded by the 1976 National Genetic Diseases Act, which combined legislation covering sickle cell and Tay-Sachs screening with provision for other disorders like cystic fibrosis, muscular dystrophy and Huntington's disease: all known to be genetic in origin. Kevles notes that by 1975 nearly half a million Americans had been screened for sickle cell trait, and tens of thousands more had been screened for Tay-Sachs or thalassemia.[19]

Eugenic sterilization and discrimination continues

On a broader scale, many of the values and practices of old-style eugenics remained in the UK and the USA throughout the 1960s and 1970s. Although disabled people were beginning to mobilize as a movement, prompting government policies to combat discrimination in both countries, people with learning disabilities or psychiatric conditions remained stigmatized and subject to coercive treatments. By this time mental health was viewed as a largely medical problem. For example, in the UK the Mental Health Act of 1959 rejected the notion of mental deficiency in favour of terms such as 'handicapped' and 'mentally subnormal'. However, as Thomson notes, the new terminology, particularly the term 'psychopath', 'enabled medical control to reach the "borderline" area lying between mental illness and deficiency, which had always been of greatest moral, social, and eugenic concern to the mental deficiency and mental hygiene lobbies'.[20]

Sterilization also continued on a considerable scale. Trombley notes that 10,545 women were sterilized during abortions in the UK between April 1968 and 1969.[21] Although a legal precedent was set against sterilization without consent in England in 1975 (which lasted until 1987), no legislation was introduced to prevent sterilization abuse. In Scotland sterilization was particularly common, often for eugenic reasons. Trombley comments that 'many local and national politicians subscribed to the notion of degeneration, and saw sterilization as a means of alleviating the problems of the modern welfare state'.[22] David Owen, then Labour Health Secretary, condoned eugenic sterilization in some circumstances, such as when girls were 'mentally subnormal and sexually vulnerable'.[23] The Conservative politician Keith Joseph also argued in a speech in 1974 that

> A high and rising proportion of children are being born to mothers least fitted to bringing up children . . . Many . . . are unmarried . . . most of them of low intelligence . . . They are producing problem children, the future unmarried mothers, delinquents, denizens of our borstals, subnormal educational establishments, prisons and hostels for drifters . . . If we do nothing the nation moves towards degeneration, however much resources we pour into preventative work . . . Proposals to extend birth control facilities to these classes of people . . . evokes entirely understandable moral opposition . . . But which is the lesser evil . . .?[24]

Eugenic sterilization also continued in American states such as California. Pfeiffer notes: 'By 1951 over 19 000 persons had been sterilised under the Californian law. In Virginia, in the institution where Carrie Buck had lived, over 4000 had been sterilised . . . Even though the law under which she was sterilised was repealed in 1968 . . . the practice in Virginia was not stopped until 1972.'[25] Trombley also argues that in 1960s America, eugenic ideas were increasing in popularity once more. He cites the case of twenty-year-old Nancy Hernandez, who was given a choice between six months in prison or probation if she agreed to be sterilized after being found guilty of the crime of being present whilst her husband smoked marijuana (the case was later overruled after the intervention of the American

Civil Liberties Union). Other similar judgments were made, all of them involving black or Hispanic people. In 1970 the sterilization rate for black women was 9 per 1,000, twice the rate of white women. Native Americans were also targeted, well into the 1970s.[26] Indeed, Trombley argues that in the late 1960s and 1970s there was a 'sterilization explosion' in the USA. A report by the Health Research Group, written by Dr Bernard Rosenfeld, found that levels of sterilization were approaching 2 million per year. It was found that physicians coerced women into having hysterectomies in order to train medical students. Rosenberg's exposure of these practices lost him his licence in California.

Other evidence suggests that poor women, many of whom were black, were being told that welfare payments would be stopped unless they agreed to be sterilized. The government did little to stop such abuses and legislation still permitted compulsory sterilization in many states throughout this decade. Even the publication of sets of guidelines in 1974 and 1978, stressing the need for informed consent, produced little change. There was considerable eugenic sentiment behind these practices. Not only were black and poor women targeted, but the 'mentally retarded' were too, a term that was loosely applied to include girls who were sexually active at a young age.

A new sociobiology

The growth of genetics also took place in the context of increasing concern about the population explosion and a racist and misogynist backlash against black and feminist activism. Scientists also became more concerned about their own role and responsibility in society, spurred, in part, by controversy about their role in the wars and the development of nuclear weapons. Kaye shows how genetic reductionism was powerfully asserted by some in response to these growing anxieties about moral disorder and social chaos. Genetic reductionism was more than just a research strategy; it was a worldview. For example, in 1970 the Committee on Science and Public Policy of the National Academy of Sciences published a survey of the current state of the life sciences, in which they were happy to view society in biological terms, to welcome abortion that reduced the number of 'unproductive' individuals and to encourage eugenics.[27]

Others took on a more Marxist agenda in response to the sense of crisis during this period. There was considerable debate, often heated and personal, between the reductionists and groups such as Science For the People, which included amongst their numbers such distinguished scientists as Stephen Jay Gould, Richard Lewontin and Richard Levins. Geneticists such as Jon Beckwith also questioned the eugenic impetus behind sickle cell screening programmes. But it was behavioural genetics and sociobiology that generated the most controversy.

Many geneticists continued to emphasize the role of inheritance in shaping behaviour, in response to what they characterized as the dogmatic environmentalism of the social sciences. Some psychiatrists and psychologists continued to conduct research into the classic concerns of eugenicists, such as schizophrenia, using old-style twin and adoption studies. Other, more infamous, studies of heredity and behaviour were also conducted around this time. Kevles discusses a study by Jacobs and colleagues of the chromosomes of male inmates of a Scottish hospital for people with 'dangerous, violent or criminal propensities', which suggested that men with two Y chromosomes (in addition to the X chromosome) might be predisposed to aggressiveness. As a result of this research an Australian man was even acquitted of murder in 1968 on the grounds that his additional Y chromosome made him prone to violence for which he could not be held responsible.[28] Although these findings were later discredited, the association between chromosomes and criminality lingers even today.

Cyril Burt and his colleagues also conducted another equally controversial study of IQ. They published results from five studies of identical twins' IQs between 1955 and 1966. They claimed that it did not matter whether the twins were raised together or apart: their IQ levels were always similar. Thus the heritability of intelligence was powerfully asserted. In 1969, the psychologist Arthur Jensen also published his famous paper in the *Harvard Review* where he argued that the lower IQs of black people compared to white people were determined in large part by genetics. He concluded that educational schemes to improve the performance of black people had therefore failed and were, indeed, doomed to failure. Richard Herrnstein also published a similar argument about class differences in IQ two years later, the same year that William Shockley famously proposed to the American Psychological Association that people of low intelligence ought to be paid to be sterilized. In practice, sterilization of inmates prior to their release from mental institutions continued on a so-called voluntary basis well into the 1970s, so these views were far from out of touch with the mood of the time.

The notion of genetic determinism of *all* aspects of human behaviour also came to prominence once more in the 1970s. E. O. Wilson's *Sociobiology*, published in 1975, applied biological explanations to every sphere of behaviour. Despite his predominant focus on non-human subjects, the implications of his work for human social relations caught the public imagination and were widely discussed (and elaborated by Wilson in his 1978 book *On Human Nature*). Wilson's work explained male dominance over women on biological grounds (maximizing gene proliferation). He also hypothesized that homosexuality was genetic in origin. But Kaye argues that Wilson was not an apologist for the status quo, as his critics vociferously claimed. Instead he laid out a reformist agenda, highly influenced by his liberal worldview, in which he advocated the harmony of culture and biology based on a new scientific morality. Genes, he argued, had some control over culture, even if cultural change had erred from the biologically correct path. In order to find this path once more, he advocated the application of altruism (enlightened self-interest): individual service to the gene pool.

Other sociobiologists continued this theme. Richard Dawkins' *The Selfish Gene*, published in 1976, shared Wilson's belief in what Kaye has termed 'the morality of the gene' and proffered a similarly reductionist and determinist account of human society. In contrast to Wilson, however, he argued that humans must be taught to be unselfish, and this would occur through the evolution of human consciousness.

These studies, alongside Burt's and Jensen's of the previous years, provoked bitter controversy within the scientific and wider public spheres. Critics chastised Wilson for giving succour to right-wing conservatives concerned with rising welfare costs and the population growth amongst the lower classes, in an echo of the old eugenics. Leon Kamin also famously debunked Burt's claims, proving his statistics to be fraudulent. When other scholars concurred, and the crime became public, various allies, including H. J. Eysenck, defended Burt, but the bulk of the psychological community distanced themselves from the hereditarian position. As Gieryn and Figert have argued, the profession engaged in a powerful 'status degrading ceremony' in order to 'restore public confidence in the trustworthiness and authority of psychologists-as-scientists'.[29] This legitimization strategy went beyond psychology, however, and also occurred in human genetics and even the life sciences as a whole. Leading advocates of the so-called environmentalists, like Kamin, mobilized alongside colleagues from genetics and allied sciences – Dobzhansky, Lewontin and Jerry Hirsh in the USA, and Steven Rose in the UK – to highlight the methodological weaknesses of these studies. Critics argued that it was wrong to transpose genetics on to heritability (i.e. to argue that if heritability was 'proven', genetic influence was too, despite the lack of causal information about genes) and that genotype and phenotype could not be separated in studies of this kind. Moreover, they charged their authors with right-wing political bias. These arguments enhanced their image as neutral scientific critics, despite the links of many to the political left. As Paul writes,

By the 1970s, the academic landscape had changed. Views that in the prior decade had been considered 'environmentalist' [were] now marked out as the opposite ... The view that genetic diversity was desirable and should be preserved had once been associated with progressive politics. At least in some circles, it now came to be identified as conservative.[30]

However, she also notes that 'the focus on the problem of heredity also unwittingly reinforced the view that hereditability estimates *mattered*'.[31]

Conclusion

This chapter demonstrates the co-evolution of eugenics and genetics during the inter- and post-war periods, up until the 1970s. Eugenic ideology also continued to exert an influence on science, medicine and social policy more broadly. In many ways the processes of reform, both scientific and social, blunted the force of eugenics. Its influence became more muted, latent and implicit. However, medical genetics grew out of eugenically inspired genetic counselling and continued to be directive even when the eugenic label had fallen out of favour. Developments in molecular biology also bolstered genetic determinism as a research method and worldview. Several leading geneticists remained at the vanguard of eugenic thinking, as others led the opposition. At the institutional level, links between genetics and eugenics in this period are also clear. Not only were funding bodies motivated by eugenic concerns, but also leading geneticists represented their profession and the eugenics movement simultaneously.

Similarly, behavioural genetics, social Darwinism and sociobiology retained and reworked eugenic ideology throughout this period. Social policy and eugenics were also intertwined, as policies and practices of sterilization clearly show. Reformed rhetoric and provision for disabled people did little to improve the position of people with learning difficulties or psychiatric disorders. The agenda of public health may have replaced overt eugenic rhetoric where screening was concerned, but the long association between public health and eugenics continued, and problems of coercion and discrimination remained.

This account challenges the tendency amongst many of the contemporary supporters of genetics to separate genetics from eugenics, or disease from social deviance. It also suggests that it is wrong to be complacent about eugenics, seeing it as confined to the beginning of the twentieth century, given its influence in the recent past. This is a useful lesson for the chapter that follows, which details contemporary developments in genetics, often termed 'the new genetics'. Whilst eugenics may be more diffuse, its legacy continues, and the apparent rift between science and social policy can be easily bridged, now as in the past. We also need to pay close attention to eugenics in the clinic, as this becomes the principal site of application of new genetic technologies, especially diagnostics.

6

The rise of the new genetics

Since the early 1970s the organized eugenics movement has been a spent force. In 1972 the American Eugenics Society became the Society for the Study of Social Biology. By 1989 the British Eugenics Society had became a small learned society called the Galton Society. But the legacy of eugenics remained in the reform eugenics and medical genetics of the post-war era. The rise of the new genetics introduced powerful techniques to splice, recombine and clone DNA, and allowed for the identification and elimination of genetic disease on an entirely new scale.

In this chapter we trace the rise of this new genetics, from the 1970s to the present, covering the Human Genome Project, genetic screening, gene therapy, cloning and the new behavioural genetics. We consider these developments in their social context, particularly the growth of the commercial sector (especially patenting), neoliberal ideals of choice and individuality, and surveillance medicine. This acts as an introduction to the remainder of the book, where we join the current debates about the social implications of these developments.

From human genetics to rDNA

By the 1970s human genetics had expanded considerably. Terminology and techniques were increasingly standardized and various subspecialties had emerged. In clinical genetics, knowledge about genetic variations and the association between genotype and phenotype (the symptoms of the genetic disorder) grew. In cytogenetics, chromosomes could be identified relatively quickly and clearly. In somatic cell genetics, techniques of cell hybridization developed and cultured fibroblasts were used in the study of genetic diseases. These developments meant that chromosome mapping and prenatal diagnosis also expanded.

The invention of recombinant DNA (rDNA) was a more revolutionary development. This enabled geneticists to splice and recombine pieces of

DNA. Enzymes could cut DNA at particular points, and the pieces could then be isolated and compared to a known piece of DNA that was radio-actively labelled. This could then be used to aid the diagnosis of genetic mutations. However, as Krimsky notes in *Genetic Alchemy*, rDNA was initially greeted with caution by the profession in the USA, where it was developed, because of fears that it might be used to create dangerous hybrid viruses or to engineer the germ-line. The community was already concerned by Paul Berg's experiments with animal tumour viruses, where he was trying to move genes in and out of animal cells in order to develop gene therapy techniques. More generally, scientists' contentious roles in the nuclear arms race and the Vietnam War meant that there was consider-able sensitivity about their professional responsibilities.

The debate about rDNA spilled out into the wider community, partly because of this ambivalence about scientists' regulatory responsibilities. In response, the American National Institutes of Health (NIH) established the Recombinant DNA Molecule Professional Advisory Committee (RAC) in 1974. Various public meetings were also organized by the NIH's Director's Advisory Committee (DAC). However, these efforts at public involvement were little more than window-dressing. The RAC was in fact keen to keep decision making within the scientific community. It proposed a voluntary moratorium on experiments with genes that code for antibiotic resistance and toxins, and restrictions on experiments involving genes for cancer or other animal viruses. But dissent was brewing beyond the bounds of the committee. This was expressed at the DAC meetings, in uni-versities and in local and state government meetings. Scientific and environmental critics of the new techniques formed the Coalition for Re-sponsible Genetic Research in 1976 and various efforts were made to introduce restrictive legislation in Congress. The media also kept up their focus on the potential applications of the new techniques, and related ef-forts of genetic engineering, including human cloning.

Ultimately the NIH moratorium was relaxed, largely because of the greater authority and wealth of the rDNA lobby, which included scientists, industrialists and government representatives. As Susan Wright has argued, leading universities and multinational pharmaceutical and chemical com-panies formed a powerful alliance that fostered genetic research and commercial development.[1] The American state actively promoted these collaborations, and fostered the small genetic engineering companies that were beginning to emerge around this time. She notes:

> By 1981 it was difficult to find a recombinant DNA practitioner who did not have a connection with private industry. Furthermore, strong business links were also formed through corporate support for

multimillion-dollar institutes, research programs and scientific departments at leading universities. Finally, the universities developed commercial interests of their own through the establishment of a variety of institutional mechanisms that would enable them to profit from the commercial application of research results.[2]

American universities began to apply for patents on the results of their genetic research. The first application was made by Stanford University in 1974 when it applied for patents on the gene-splicing work of Cohen and colleagues. The American government changed patenting legislation to support the universities' rights to patent the processes for making novel organisms and the organisms themselves. This new commercial environment fostered secrecy and distrust amongst the genetics community. But at the same time, research was proceeding on an international scale, with scientists from different countries collaborating on research projects. Geneticists also began to 'hype' their results more effectively. Advocates of recombinant DNA research skilfully promoted its benefits. For example, much was made of the discovery by an international team of scientists in 1978 of the gene that produces haemoglobin.

By the end of the 1970s the rDNA controversy no longer focused on laboratory biohazards, but turned to the commercial development of the technology, particularly the large-scale growth of protein products such as insulin and interferon. Corporations' safety protocols and patenting policies came under review and concerns were raised about professional scientists profiting from their research. However, the media tended to present these developments as 'good news' for human health. Further relaxation of the NIH guidelines followed.

Krimsky notes that, at the same time, efforts were also made to increase public participation in the RAC, and a network of Institutional Biosafety Committees, which included public representatives, was established.[3] Local community groups negotiated with big firms and universities engaged in rDNA research, and environmentalists continued to lobby for controls on the release of potentially dangerous organisms into the environment. Jeremy Rifkin and colleagues focused in particular on the misuses of genetic engineering. He published a book on the issue with Ted Howard which drew its title from the religious concerns about the new techniques: *Who Shall Play God?*

Early gene therapy and embryo research

Cloning and gene therapy were amongst the most controversial techniques to be developed in this period. Animal cloning techniques had been developed in the early 1960s, to produce uniform stock from early embryos. Early embryonic cells could also be manipulated to introduce foreign DNA. The first transgenic mouse of 1982 contained a growth hormone gene from the rat. Other forms of gene therapy involved molecular cloning, where DNA was inserted into yeast or bacteria to multiply. As Martin notes, initially the focus of this research was on classical genetic disorders such as thalassemia. The aim was to alter patients' cells either by removing them, adding 'good' genes and reinfusing them into the patient's body (ex vivo therapy) or by directly injecting the genes into the patient's body (in vivo therapy). These techniques were pursued until the early 1980s, when controversy about the ethics of gene therapy had a decisive impact on this research.

Martin tells the story of Dr Martin Cline, a well-known clinician from the University of California at Los Angeles, who performed gene therapy on patients in Italy and Israel in 1980 without the approval of his Institutional Review Board, an important monitor of research ethics that had to give approval prior to consideration by the RAC. This sparked considerable protest about gene therapy, which, in turn, prompted an inquiry by the President's Commission for the Study of Ethical Problems in Medicine and Biomedical and Behavioural Research, whose findings were reported in *Splicing Life*, an important document in the regulation of genetic therapy. As Martin notes,

> The Commission's report was important in making a distinction between the neo-eugenic idea of altering future generations, which it called germ line therapy, and the medical use of gene transfer directed solely at treating the non-reproductive cells of an individual patient, which it labelled somatic gene therapy. The Commission believed that germ line therapy was unethical and should not be allowed, but it felt that it was acceptable to proceed with the development of somatic therapy for life threatening genetic diseases . . . This distinction has subsequently played a key role in helping legitimise somatic therapy as little more than a conventional medical intervention and has shaped all subsequent debates about the ethics of gene therapy.[4]

The dominant research efforts (still only pursued by fewer than ten research laboratories in the USA), which focused on single gene disorders (mainly of the blood), reached a dead-end in the mid-1980s, mainly due to technical difficulties with gene transfer. But, as Martin argues, this set the stage for the later, successful, attempts at gene transfer by W. French Anderson, who drew on gene therapy's redefinition as an experimental medical procedure, which was carefully regulated and ethically acceptable.

Martin shows how Anderson developed a range of professional and commercial alliances in order to conduct his research into gene therapy. Initially he focused on adenosine deaminase (ADA) deficiency – a rare disorder of the immune system which is fatal in childhood. Anderson won regulatory approval for his proposal to conduct a preclinical trial, only after changing his approach to the transfer of genetic markers into the white blood cells of patients who had bone marrow transplants to treat leukaemia. As Martin argues, this presaged a rapid expansion of the gene therapy field in the 1990s, key features of which were commercial development in the biotechnology industry, a reconstitution of the notion of genetic disease to include common conditions such as cancer and heart disease, and a change in gene therapy from a surgical procedure to a drug therapy.

Similar political, commercial and scientific alliances characterized the development of a limited framework of regulatory control of in vitro fertilization and embryo research in the UK during the 1980s (a framework that formed the basis for regulation in other countries, including the USA). Edwards, Steptoe and Purdy's development of in vitro fertilization (IVF), culminating in the birth of Louise Brown in 1978, was widely publicized and emulated during the early part of the 1980s. As Mike Mulkay notes in *The Embryo Research Debate: Science and the Politics of Reproduction*, it became the topic of intense public scrutiny in the UK in the 1980s, prompting the Warnock Committee's investigation and report of 1984, which in turn sparked wider interest in the morality of research into human embryos. A long period of public and parliamentary debate followed this report, which was to result in the Human Fertilisation and Embryology Bill (HFEB) of 1990.

Mulkay tells how the pro-research lobby triumphed over the critics of embryo research in the context of a growing demand for infertility treatment, which opened the way for embryo experimentation. A strong coalition of scientists, doctors, parliamentarians and birth control campaigners lobbied in support of embryo research. The profession also established a Voluntary Licensing Authority to underline its ethical and responsible practice, and to emphasize the role of IVF and embryo research in the prevention of disability, specifically the reduction in genetic disorders (through the implantation of healthy embryos in the mother's womb), in contrast to the ethically dubious alteration or replacement of human genes. As Mulkay comments,

> This representation of embryo research, guaranteed by the authority of the scientific establishment, appealed directly to that subtle combination of progressive and conservative ideals that define the middle

ground of British politics. The pro research lobby succeeded because the majority of Labour progressives and Conservative moderates were unable to resist a programme of continuous scientific development which, so they believed, had been shown to offer substantial social progress without requiring any significant alterations to social values or essential social relationships.[5]

This, alongside related developments in gene therapy and cloning, set the stage for a considerable expansion of IVF and embryo research in the coming decade.

Early clinical genetics

At the same time as these public debates about gene therapy and embryo research were being held, developments in clinical genetics were also moving on apace. The ability to distinguish, and in some cases map, particular genes to locations on the chromosomes meant that geneticists could search out and identify mutant genes.

In *The Gene Wars*, Cook-Deegan describes one of the earliest examples of this – the work on sickle cell disease by Yuet Wai Kan and A. M. Dozy at the University of California. This team identified a particular segment of DNA, called a marker, which was associated with the sickle cell gene in families of North African descent. They could then track this marker through the generations to see if children would develop the disease. Another landmark development was the discovery by Mark Skolnick and colleagues at the University of Utah of the gene for haemachromatosis – a disease that involves high levels of iron in the blood and associated problems with liver and heart function. The team built on previous research that had linked haemachromatosis to other cell surface markers, studying in depth the DNA of families with the disease. They concluded that the disease involved a recessive pattern of inheritance. The group proceeded to direct analysis of the DNA variations in order to find differences among individuals in families and thus locate the problem gene.

Cook-Deegan tells how genetic researchers then began to develop techniques to construct a linkage map based on genetic markers. Raymond White, for example, studied the inheritance of naturally occurring variations in DNA and their associations with disease genes. If markers were consistently inherited alongside disease genes then the gene could be pinpointed to a particular chromosome. Biotechnology companies, such as Collaborative Research Inc., also took up this approach. In 1987 the company announced a genetic linkage map which, although incomplete, was the catalyst for yet more mapping and an important precursor to the Human Genome Project.

As Cook-Deegan notes, 'with maps in hand, gene hunts became highly competitive races'.[6] By 1985 researchers had identified markers for the genes responsible for Huntington's disease (1983), Duchenne muscular dystrophy (1983), polycystic kidney disease (1985), retinoblastoma (1985) and cystic fibrosis (1985). The actual genes were more difficult to find because of the painstaking search through DNA that this involved, but several high-profile successes did occur, notably the identification of the Huntington's gene in 1993, and the cystic fibrosis gene in 1989, only four years after the marker was found. Other disease genes were more difficult to pinpoint because of the clinical heterogeneity and multiple involvement of genes therein. One example of this is Alzheimer's disease. In 1987 two research groups linked Alzheimer's to a region of chromosome 21, while others linked it to chromosomes 19 and 24, suggesting that Alzheimer's as a category involved clinically similar disorders caused by different genetic defects.

The Human Genome Project

Surprisingly, as Cook-Deegan notes, these early efforts at human gene mapping did not grow into the Human Genome Project (HGP). Instead, they were incorporated at a later stage. The HGP developed first from other studies of the structure of DNA, many involving non-human subjects. Researchers in these fields developed physical maps of DNA, which were to bridge the gap between linkage maps and DNA sequences. The first 'gene libraries' were based on cloned DNA from an entire organism. Fragments of the DNA were copied and stored. Probes could then be used to search out particular pieces of DNA and the genes identified could be mapped, or physically located on the chromosome. Other developments in DNA sequencing also preceded the HGP. The HGP grew, in part, from research into the genetic effects of radiation, as the US national laboratories realigned themselves towards the study of human health via genetics. The development of another technique, the polymerase chain reaction, allowed researchers to copy DNA without having to use bacteria or other organisms to clone it. By the late 1980s various automated sequencing devices were also on the market, speeding up the sequencing process considerably.

These commercial developments were not, however, smooth. Instead they were marked by considerable tension and rivalry between academia and commerce, and between different nations. This was to continue throughout the Human Genome Project. Scientists' commercial interests and roles were also problematic, with high-profile figures such as Walter Gilbert moving between the private and university sector, and initiating various attempts to privatise gene mapping and sequencing.

In 1986 the American Department of Energy announced the Human Genome Initiative, based on $5.3 million of pilot projects to develop the critical resources and techniques necessary for a project to map and sequence the human genome. In the following years, various levels of American bureaucracy investigated and pronounced on the plans for such a scheme. International meetings were held by scientists where they also debated the pros and cons of a large mapping and sequencing project. Concerns were expressed about siphoning off funds for other research and the large cost of such a programme. Scientists also set up the International Human Genome Organization in an effort to co-ordinate research, which was also developing in Europe and Japan in particular. After considerable debate within the scientific community and between the NIH and the Department of Energy, the Human Genome Project's remit changed from a focus on sequencing to mapping. Research into non-human subjects was also incorporated, as was a focus on specific genetic defects of medical interest. The proposals for the HGP broadened, to command sufficient support from the scientific community in the USA and abroad.

James Watson was appointed as the head of the NIH genome office in 1988. Despite considerable debate within the American government and the scientific press about the growing budget of the project, the HGP began in 1990 with the NIH and Department of Energy spending a total of $86.7 million in that year. An international effort was under way to sequence the entire human genome, estimated at three billion base-pairs, and to discover the estimated 100,000 genes therein. Italy announced that it would join the programme in 1987, as did the UK, whose programme began in April 1989 as a three-year project, initially focusing on automation and areas of DNA of special interest. By 1990 the Wellcome Trust had made a major commitment to research co-ordinated by the Human Genome Organization (HUGO). Russian and French genome programmes also emerged, as did smaller projects in Germany and Denmark. Japan also became involved.

Private initiatives were especially important in Europe, notably in France, where the privately organized Centre for the Study of Human Polymorphism (CEPH), in alliance with the private muscular dystrophy association, AFM, set up Genethon, based on large amounts of money raised through telethons. In the UK, two important charities, the Wellcome Trust and the Imperial Cancer Research Fund, also financed

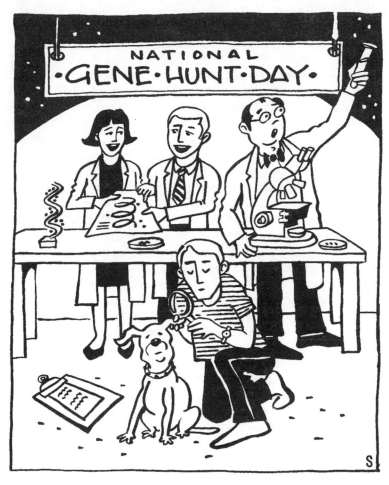

genome research, with the Wellcome's contribution overtaking the British government's in 1993.

Given the growing commercial interest in genetics throughout the 1970s, and the international competition inevitable in a project with such implications for pharmaceutical and technological treatment and diagnosis of disease, it is not surprising that the HGP and associated sequencing efforts remained controversial. It involved numerous struggles over ownership in particular. Watson's resignation as director of the NIH Genome Office in 1991 occurred because of a prolonged battle with the director of the NIH, Bernadine Healy. Healy oversaw an investigation into Watson's financial holdings at a time when the two disagreed vigorously over the patenting policy of the NIH (with Healy in favour of patenting and Watson against). As Sir Walter Bodmer, the director of the British Imperial Cancer Research Fund and a prominent figure in HUGO, acknowledged in *The Wall Street Journal*, 'the issue [of ownership] is at the heart of everything we do'.[7]

A massive global project developed in both the public and commercial realms, with considerable ramifications for the identification and treatment of genetic diseases. Funding for the HGP was again increased, to $169.1 million in the fiscal year 1993, in response to Craig Venter's establishment of a private company, Celera Inc., which planned to utilize a different, less precise, technique called whole genome shotgun sequencing. Celera aimed to sequence the genome in three years, for a cost of $300 million, a fraction of the cost of the HGP. The company also planned to patent the genes of interest and to market the whole genome on a subscription basis to genetic researchers. The HGP responded by setting up a public database and condemned patenting practices. President Bill Clinton and Prime Minister Tony Blair even issued a vague statement outlining their commitment to open data, whilst Clinton elaborated his support for patent protection to encourage financial investment in science elsewhere. But his caveat was not enough to prevent the stock markets from reacting, knocking billions off the value of biotechnology shares. The economic reality of genetics meant that political and scientific leaders had to walk a tightrope between public interest and commercial gain. The leaders of the HGP also had to negotiate with Celera, albeit reluctantly.

Despite their talk of 'synergy' between the private and public genome projects, the Wellcome Trust and the NIH moved to increase their funding in order to speed up their completion of the genome, and announced that they would produce a working draft by the end of 2001 and a complete map by 2003. But the drafts of the estimated 30,000 genes that are thought to make up the human genome (a considerably smaller number than initially predicted) were completed earlier still. In February 2001, *Nature* published the initial analysis of the sequence generated by the HGP and *Science* published Celera's draft.

Francis Collins noted at the White House press conference announcing the two maps that most of the sequencing had in fact been done in the previous fifteen months. This joint announcement is symbolic of the private–public relationship around the genome. Celera and the HGP are bound together in mutual antagonism. Tensions exist about ownership and standards, but the two groups must collaborate when it comes to public relations and replicability. The HGP aims to develop what it calls 'an entire reference genome', in contrast to private-sector projects that focus on lucrative regions of the genome. The HGP's policy of open data contrasts with the fee-paying service offered by private companies such as Celera, but the

HGP argues that its data are fundamental to the construction of these private maps. This makes for continued tension between the private and public sectors – especially where patenting is concerned, as we shall discuss shortly – but the overarching rhetoric emphasizes public–private partnership, as the following quote from the HGP information website illustrates:

> An important feature of this project is the federal government's long-standing dedication to the transfer of technology to the private sector. By licensing technologies to private companies and awarding grants for innovative research, the project is catalyzing the multibillion-dollar US biotechnology industry and fostering the development of new medical applications.[8]

In the press conference to announce the working draft of the genome, Clinton and Blair emphasized this public–private partnership, and characterized government's role as a facilitator and moderator of technological developments to ensure that the technology was put to the common good rather than abused to 'make men their own creator', as Blair put it, or to invade privacy and foster discrimination. They also talked of its historic significance, Clinton describing it as the most important map ever produced, illustrating the commonality of humanity.

But it is the commercial potential of the genome that is of most interest to western governments. As Venter noted at the same press conference, P. E. Biosystems invested over $1 billion in Celera's enterprise. IBM, Compaq, DuPont and major pharmaceutical companies are all investing in the area, and many smaller companies are now conducting research into genetic data and their applications. 'For-profit genomics' focuses on diagnostic technologies and drug developments, many of them at an exploratory stage. As Malakoff and Service comment, the stock values of such companies are often based on market potential rather than actual innovations.[9] The future of gene brokers like Celera is uncertain, as public databases grow. The products of companies like Millenium, who are engaged in developing drugs to treat multifactorial diseases, could take many years to develop. However, 'toolmakers' who sell sequencing technologies are beginning to make a profit, and DNA chip technology that enables companies rapidly to screen large numbers of genes may well speed up drug development times.

Gene patenting

Commercial interests are apparent throughout genomics, as the patenting of genes shows. In 1998 the US Patent Office received more than 13,000 biotechnology patent applications and had granted 2,000, including patents on 85 mice, three rabbits, a sheep and a cow. Amongst the most troubling applications is one by John Gearhart, a researcher at Johns Hopkins University, who has applied for a patent on his procedure to use cells from aborted embryos to grow spare human parts (he is backed by Geron Corporation).

Patents have also been taken out on the DNA on indigenous peoples, and on the DNA of people with rare genetic disorders. Groups representing indigenous people have protested about the practice and called for an end to 'biopiracy'. Although these controversies meant that the Human Genetic Diversity Project did not become a formal project, samples continue to be collected across the world, and the European Commission funds work on the 'biological history of European populations'. Some relatives involved in genetic studies have also protested about the use of their children's DNA. For example, relatives of children with Canavan's syndrome collaborated with researchers at the Miami Children's Hospital in the USA, by providing tissue samples to aid the development of genetic tests, only to find that the scientists and the hospitals they worked for went on to patent the gene, restricting access to carrier testing and further study of the disease.

Gene patents do not inevitably restrict research and testing. They do not need to involve exclusive licensing agreements, as in the cystic fibrosis gene test patented by the universities of Toronto and Michigan, which charge a token $2 per test. Nor do they need to restrict academic research. Johns Hopkins University researchers Vogelstein, and Kinzler and colleagues have a patent on a technique to identify genes involved in disease which authorizes free use of the technology by academics.[10] However, patenting for profit is big business. Amongst the disease genes that have been patented for profit are a gene involved in Alzheimer's (patented to Duke University and licensed to Glaxo) and a gene involved in obesity (patented to Millenium Pharmaceuticals, licensed to Hoffman LaRoche). Myriad Genetics and the University of Utah own a patent for the hereditary breast and ovarian cancer genes BRCA-1 and BRCA-2 and have developed a test that costs about £1,500. They are currently trying to enforce the patent to stop other hospitals across the world from conducting their own tests and to force them to use the Myriad test. The British government has negotiated with the Cancer Research Campaign, which owns the European patent on the BRCA-2 gene test, to allow free testing on the National Health Service, but this is the exception rather than the rule in the global marketplace of genomics.

Large corporations are also buying up small biotechnology start-up companies, and venture capitalists, including Bill Gates, are investing heavily in the biotechnology industry: Gates is a major investor in

Darwin Molecular, which holds a patent on a gene thought to be involved in premature ageing and responsible for a rare disorder called Werner's syndrome. The activities of Celera give some clue as to future commercial practice in this sector. The company offers fee-paying clients access to a gene database based on its research. Although this competes with the free, publicly available HGP sequence, it remains commercially viable. Celera has several major subscribers, including universities, research institutions and biotechnology and pharmaceutical companies. Celera has also bought up various add-on databases to enhance its commercial appeal, with the aim of becoming a 'one-stop shopping place for life-science researchers', according to James Peck, a Celera manager.[11]

The HGP's massive public database, Genebank, aims to undermine this commodification of life. Other public–private partnerships, such as that between ten large pharmaceutical companies and the Wellcome Trust single nucleotide polymorphism (SNP) mapping project, also intend to make their map publicly available, and to do so they will patent (to prevent others from patenting the same information), but not enforce the patents. Patients' groups such as PXE International (pseudoxanthoma elasticum is a rare genetic condition that causes the skin, eyes and arteries to harden) have also begun to make joint patent applications with the research team that identified the gene involved in the condition, in order to ensure that any tests developed are widely available and cheap.[12]

But the sheer scale of commercial patenting activity cannot be stemmed by efforts such as these. As Bobrow and Thomas note, many thousands of patents on human DNA have been filed and granted. The 31,000 genes identified in the working draft of the genome, although well short of the 100,000 initially predicted, are nevertheless a large number of genes with significant commercial potential. Gene patenting is also likely to thrive as the regulatory context is lax, as Bobrow and Thomas comment:

> In the absence of serious legislative action, policy has more or less evolved through dialogue within a limited circle of participants. Commercial interests, which are well represented to the patent offices, have not been counter-balanced by those who represent the broader public interest. The result has been an innate tendency for the patent system to 'creep' in the direction of extending patentability to biotechnology inventions for which the thresholds for novelty, inventiveness and utility have been lowered.[13]

Developments in pharmacogenomics, particularly the lucrative market for gene-based treatments for multifactorial conditions like cancer that are the holy grail of this sector, can only intensify this scramble to commodify disease.

Gene therapy and pharmacogenomics

Although in May 2000 gene therapy was reported to have been successfully used by French researchers to treat two babies with severe
autoimmunodeficiency (SCID), by providing a normal copy of the defective gene through a retrovirus delivered to the patient's stem cells,[14] this
area of research has been blighted by the death of clinical subjects, their
subsequent concealment by the researchers involved and considerable
concern about conflicts of interest arising from researchers' ownerships of
stocks in the companies developing these techniques.

In September 1999, and the months that followed, *The Washington
Post* revealed a catalogue of cases where gene therapy researchers had
failed to report the deaths of volunteers to the NIH, as required by federal
law. An inquiry by Congress revealed that this practice was widespread.
The use of potentially toxic viruses as delivery systems was partly to
blame, but many of these deaths remain unexplained. This has led to the
suspension of numerous gene therapy trials in the USA, some voluntarily,
and some at the behest of the Food and Drug Administration (FDA).

A more recent and potentially lucrative area of research is that of
pharmacogenetics, which aims to establish 'personal pharmacogenetic
profiles' based on patients' genotypes, and to understand and treat
common multifactorial diseases such as cancer or heart disease with drugs
based on genetic knowledge. Pharmaceutical companies are pouring vast
amounts of money into the genomic approach to drug development, and
studies of the genetic variations that determine the suitability of drugs
for particular patients, in order to prevent adverse drug reactions. For
example, particularly in Scandinavia, pharmacogenomic testing for the
CYP2D6 genotype is used to aid dose selection for drugs used to treat psychiatric illnesses.[15]

One of the most high-profile examples of pharmacogenomic research
companies is that of deCode Genetics, which has obtained a licence from
the Icelandic government to establish a nationwide database incorporating
health, genetic and genealogical information on the whole population (individuals must opt out through a complex procedure to be removed from
the database). The deCode case is another instance of government and
commercial synergy, with deCode having exclusive rights to the data, but
the power to enter into commercial agreements with other companies, and
the government welcoming the boost to the Icelandic economy that these
developments will bring.

The considerable hubbub around the potential developments in this
field must, of course, be treated with caution, given its role in boosting

share prices. The complexity of disease and the potential side-effects of new drug developments are serious problems. But on a longer timescale, pharmacogenomics could mean that more and more people are subject to genetic screening. Insurance companies and employers in particular are likely to be very interested in the results of such tests, as we shall discuss later. As the focus shifts to common diseases, people with rare genetic disorders may lose out. Pharmacogenomics could also intensify the move towards a two-tier health care system, where people who are not 'genetically suitable' for particular drugs are simply excluded from treatment because there is no profit to be made from developing alternative drugs for such a small population.

Another worrying development in the area of genetic therapy is the re-invigoration of germ-line engineering in the genomic era. Developments in reproductive medicine and genetic research could be combined to modify the sperm or egg cells before fertilization or the undifferentiated cells of the early embryo to introduce genes that will be passed through the generations. This technique is already used on laboratory animals and somatic gene therapy has been attempted on human embryos. Although there are numerous obstacles to such practices, which require large numbers of eggs and may result in deleterious combinations of genes that cannot be known in advance, various well-known geneticists and support groups have begun to call for the development of the technique, and there is no international ban on the practice. The blurred boundary between treatment or therapy and enhancement of physical and mental characteristics raises further concerns about the potential uses of this technology.

Towards reproductive cloning

Developments in nuclear transfer have also opened the way for reproductive cloning, another eugenics dream. Dolly the sheep was created in 1997, the result of fusing a mammary gland cell from a dead sheep with an enucleated egg. President Clinton announced a moratorium on federal funding for human cloning using such a technique shortly afterwards. But a US company, Advanced Cell Technology, recently claimed to have used similar techniques to produce cloned human embryos of between four and six cells. The aim of scientists working in this field is to develop the technique to produce personalized spare parts for future treatments of illnesses and diseases like Parkinson's and dementia: so-called therapeutic cloning. The UK has recently relaxed restrictions on this process so that it can be used to create embryonic stem cells, although the embryos must be destroyed after fourteen days. Not only do these developments raise concerns about the commodification of the body, in the form of donor embryos and cloned tissue and organs; these techniques could be adopted in the pursuit of reproductive cloning. Although this is currently illegal in countries such as the UK, no worldwide ban exists. The large numbers of discarded eggs required to make a clone, considerable foetal loss during pregnancy and after birth, and frequent genetic abnormalities in the resulting clones, severely restrict the potential of human cloning. But a growing band of scientists and doctors aim to develop the technique nevertheless.

The first to proclaim his intentions was Dr Richard Seed; he was quickly followed by researchers at an infertility clinic in Korea, which claimed in 1998 to have successfully cloned a human but destroyed the embryo because of ethical qualms. An obscure cult called the Raelians also announced its intention to clone a human embryo, claiming to have 50 women willing to take part in the experiment and an American couple with a dead child's DNA to be cloned. And in 2001 a team of fertility experts in Italy, Israel and the USA announced their intentions to produce the first human clone. Unlike Seed or the Raelains, Professor Severino Antinori is an established figure, currently president of the Italian Society of Reproductive Medicine and head of a number of IVF clinics in Rome. Although the possibilities of reproductive cloning are remote, it would be foolish to ignore these efforts to develop the technique in humans.

The growth of clinical genetics

Many significant disease genes have been identified since the beginning of the Human Genome Project. Although not all of these have been under its auspices, it is undoubtedly true that the HGP has made a massive contribution to disease gene identification. More than a dozen disease genes were identified by researchers using the HGP database in the year prior to the announcement of the draft map. Gene tests have also developed rapidly in this period. The website of Genetests™ (www.genetests.org), a directory of worldwide laboratories offering gene tests, lists 819 diseases for which gene tests are available, either commercially or as part of research, as of July 2001.

Gene testing tends to fall under five main categories. It can be diagnostic, predictive, prenatal, postnatal or carrier testing. *Diagnostic* testing is used to confirm or rule out a suspected genetic disorder, where the patient already has apparent symptoms. *Predictive* testing, on the other hand, involves tests prior to the onset of particular symptoms. It can be performed for late onset disorders like Huntington's disease (where no treatment is available) or for other diseases such as familial breast and ovarian cancer, where it gives an estimate of the person's susceptibility to cancer, given that environmental factors also play a part in the condition. This means that people who are highly susceptible can modify their lifestyle or engage in regular screening (although, in this example, there is thought to be little benefit of repeated mammography in younger women).

As Marteau and Croyle note of the UK in particular, 'at present, most of the genetic tests that are carried out are reproductive tests which provide information about the chances of genetic disorders in future children'.[16] *Prenatal* testing is currently available for families with a history of genetic disorders like cystic fibrosis, Huntington's disease and Fragile-X syndrome in most molecular genetic laboratories in the UK and the USA. Many of these diseases are very rare, and are becoming rarer as prenatal testing is offered to more pregnant women. For example, the birth frequency of Duchenne muscular dystrophy in the UK had fallen from 1 in 6,000 when genetic counselling began, to 1 in 9,000 in the UK by 1999.[17]

Prenatal testing usually takes place at between ten and fifteen weeks of pregnancy, depending on the method used (chorionic villus sampling can be performed earlier than amniocentesis). This can be used to test women at risk of a genetic disorder because of a family history of the disease. Rarely, treatment can be offered to mitigate the effects of the disorder, either in the womb, during delivery or immediately after the baby is born. More usually abortion is offered. In the UK there is no upper time limit on abortions because of 'serious handicap'. In the USA it tends to be left to individual physicians to decide on the viability of a foetus, and state legislatures are prohibited by federal law from banning abortion for non-viable foetuses (although there are other ways in which they can restrict and delay provision). The time delay in receiving results of antenatal tests (or, in the case of the USA, other requirements for delayed decision making) means that abortions for foetal abnormality are usually performed in the second trimester.

Prenatal screening is applied to a larger population, but it is less common for genetic disorders. Although many in the profession favour its expansion – the NIH is pushing forward cystic fibrosis screening in the USA, for example – screening can also be unpopular because of concerns about its efficacy given ethnic variations, as well as its costs. The disintegration of publicly funded national health services also limits its viability. However, some screening programmes are available to certain groups who are thought to be particularly susceptible to a genetic disease because of their ethnic origins, for example. The thalassaemia screening service in the UK is one such programme.

Postnatal genetic tests are performed on newborns thought to be at risk of a genetic disorder, and postnatal screening tests all babies for genetic conditions like PKU, most of which can be treated. Newborn screening is mandated by law in the USA for certain genetic diseases. All states test for PKU but other tests vary from state to state. States variously test for congenital hypothyroid disease, galactosaemia, maple syrup urine disease, homocystinuria, biothnidase deficiency, sickle cell anaemia, congenital adrenal hyperplasia, cystic fibrosis and tyrosinaemia. As Clayton comments,

> One consequence of having a well-developed infrastructure for newborn screening for PKU, however, is that it has made it much easier to think about adding screening for other disorders to these programs . . . The pressure to add tests for other disorders is ever present. But even the most thoughtful analyses of proposals to screen for new disorders generally fail to address adequately the question of why a particular test should be added to the armamentarium.[18]

In the UK, postnatal screening for PKU and other related disorders is in place and considered to be cost effective. Neonatal screening for other conditions such as Duchenne muscular dystrophy and cystic fibrosis is more controversial because of potential difficulties with false negative results, and lack of proven benefit of early diagnosis, but the British government recently announced that it would go ahead with plans to establish a national neonatal screening programme for cystic fibrosis.

Carrier testing identifies people who are carriers for particular genetic disorders, but who are not themselves affected. The test is used to inform people of their carrier status prior to conception or marriage in some cases (for example, in the Ashkenazi Jewish community in the USA and UK, where a carrier test for Tay-Sachs disease can be used).

In the UK, genetic tests for the most serious genetic disorders are mainly provided through regional genetics services. During the 1980s clinical molecular genetics laboratories were set up in most British regional genetic centres in order to provide a diagnostic service. By 1988 a professional group, the Clinical Molecular Genetics Society (CMGS), had been formed. The clinics are regulated via a variety of bodies including a quality assurance agency, established by the CMGS. They are now operated by an independent body that provides accredited training for staff, who are then registered by one of several national registration boards, depending on their specialism. Laboratories must also be accredited and the government's Advisory Committee on Genetic Testing oversees the safe and ethical use of genetic tests. NHS regional genetics centres are multi-disciplinary and counselling is offered to all clients, who are referred by their general practitioner or another consultant, such as a paediatrician. Centres collaborate, but a national strategy has yet to emerge since the introduction of the internal market in the NHS. Instead collaboration tends to occur via professional bodies and consortiums formed to oversee and co-ordinate research or to conduct audits of practices.

In the USA, genetic testing services are provided by genetic clinics attached to universities or set up by private companies, most of which are run for profit. Clients are usually referred by their physician, and clinics performing clinical tests must be licensed under the Clinical Laboratory Improvement Act/Amendment 1988 (CLIA), although this provides no specific guidance for genetic tests. Because of the patenting laws in the USA, these laboratories are restricted in the tests they may perform. Costs vary from less than $100 to more than $2,000, depending on the complexity of the test, the strategy for testing, the number of individuals tested and the type of specimen taken. The American government has funded considerable research into the social and ethical aspects of testing (for example, the now disbanded ELSI, part of the Human Genome Project) but there is no federal committee dedicated to addressing genetic testing. The Task Force on Genetic Testing did make various recommendations, including the need for organizations to establish the efficacy of proposed tests. The Food and Drug Administration reviews tests marketed as products, but those marketed as services are not reviewed by the FDA.

The speed with which many of these genetic tests and screening programmes have been developed belies some of the very real difficulties with characterizing genetic diseases, many of which are highly complex, involving a range of genes or genotypes whose impact on the symptoms and severity of the disease is not well understood. Concerns have also been raised about the lack of informed consent involved in screening programmes and about inadequate or overly directive counselling, particularly when it is performed by obstetricians as opposed to genetic counsellors. The ramifications of positive tests for wider family members, especially when children are tested and their results give information about their parents' genetic status, have also led many to criticize the proliferation of genetic testing without adequate forethought about its ethical implications. And the substitution of genetic diagnosis for proper care and support of people who are sick and disabled is raised by critics of these new technologies. We will explore all of these issues in more depth in the forthcoming chapters.

From behavioural genetics to behavioural genomics

Parallel to developments in clinical and molecular genetics, behavioural genetics has continued to evolve, applying new molecular techniques to the study of homosexuality, alcoholism, IQ and criminality, amongst other traits. Psychiatric genetics has also blossomed. Twin and adoption studies continue to be controversial, and linkage studies based on DNA analysis to identify particular markers in families that are affected by disorders such as depression are also problematic because of difficulties with replicating the findings in other studies. Perhaps the most notorious of these is Dean Hamer's study of the 'gay gene', where he claimed to have identified a section of DNA on the X chromosome shared by gay brothers. But as Lehrman points out, his study did not involve any control groups, his subjects were not representative of the gay community and his results have not been replicated.[19] Animal studies, on aggression in mice, for example, have also failed to provide definitive evidence of behavioural genetic traits.

But the fanfare about the potential of psychiatric genomics continues. The media are often blamed for this hype, but it is the profession who lead the way. Promoting a sophisticated argument about the complexity of behaviour, emphasizing multi-gene systems and environmental influences, they nevertheless continue to stress the reliability of findings from twin and adoption studies which show that 'genetic variation makes a substantial contribution to phenotypic variation for all behavioral domains'[20] and claim that 'the human genome sequence will revolutionize psychology and psychiatry' and increase tolerance of psychiatric and behavioural disorder. As we will go on to discuss more fully in the next chapter, while we accept that genes do have a role in behaviour, we believe that the claims of behavioural genetics are wildly overstated. The interrelation between thousands of genes interacting with complex environmental, familial and social processes is very hard to chart. Intervening to make any difference via genetic medicine will be impossible for the foreseeable future.

The racism and elitism of the old eugenics continues to be acceptable to a minority of scientists with an interest in behavioural genetics, and it finds many supporters in the right-wing elements of society at large. The publication of *The Bell Curve* in 1994 by Richard Herrnstein and Charles Murray sparked a furore about their predicted dysgenesis of the USA due to the high fertility rates of what they called the 'cognitive underclass'[21] and their suggestion that black people are less intelligent than whites, but it gained many notable supporters. As Lind comments, 'the fortuitous appearance of *The Bell Curve* provided conservatives with a useful rationale for a policy of abolishing welfare that they already favoured'.[22] More recently, James Watson even argued that women ought to be permitted to abort a foetus if it were known to be homosexual.[23] Evolutionary psychology has also come to prominence in recent years, pioneered by media-friendly academics like Steven Pinker and Helena Cronin. Writers from this tradition resurrect the old sociobiological lines that women are genetically programmed to be homemakers and offer evolutionary explanations for many human behaviours, including rape, infanticide and President Clinton's sexual philandering. As we shall argue in the next chapter, although it is easy to scoff at these kinds of theory, their media profile is high because they offer simplistic solutions to complex problems; solutions that further reinforce the genetic determinism of human genomics.

Eugenics old and new

Today's genomics is obviously very different from the eugenics of the past – in its technological and commercial sophistication and scale, in particular – but it is not possible to draw neat divisions between the past and the present, as some contemporary advocates of genetics maintain. Throughout this book we have shown that in the past eugenics was a feature of democratic as well as totalitarian regimes. In its heyday it involved many professionals and had broad public support, and it was far from being simply biased pseudo-science. The focus may have shifted to abortion rather than sterilization or euthanasia, and to disease rather than social deviancy, but there are fine lines between these approaches. Nor is the liberal rhetoric of individual rights and informed choice the reality of many people's experience of genetic services. Even as an ideal it is flawed, as it pays too little attention to the social circumstances in which people make choices, and to the ramifications of those choices for wider society.

Although anti-discrimination legislation has been introduced in both the USA (1990) and the UK (1996) to strengthen the rights of disabled people, and the old-style mental institutions have nearly all closed in favour of community care, discrimination and stigmatization of disabled people continues, in the health service and beyond. Sterilization, enforced contraception and discrimination over access to treatment remain. As Pfeiffer notes, courts in the USA can still compel compulsory sterilization in some states, and restrict the rights of people with learning difficulties and mental disabilities to marry, and children can be removed from disabled parents with disabilities, including low IQs, hearing and speech impairment, and even epilepsy.[24] In both countries, disabled children and adults are still left to die when treatments could be administered, and disabled women are often greeted with shock and disbelief when they express a wish not to abort when genetic testing predicts a disabled child.

People with genetic disorders in their families have also found themselves unable to obtain insurance and employment, despite a hotchpotch of legislation and codes of practice supposedly designed to prevent such a situation. And the intensification of high-tech forms of surveillance such as forensic and biomedical databases may well herald new forms of biomedical control of criminal propensity.

The rise of political neoliberalism in this period, with its emphasis on individuality and enterprise, also chimes with the new forms of genetic surveillance that have emerged in the wake of the Human Genome Project. People are increasingly cast as responsible for their own health and welfare, and the state takes on the role of overseer and provider of opportunity. Although it is often argued that regulation cannot move quickly enough to deal with technological advance, the slowness of regulation is a deliberate strategy to open up possibilities for technology and commercial expansion.

A whole new ethical industry has developed alongside genomics, which often tends towards pushing the boundaries of acceptability and advocating controversial practices such as germ-line engineering. More critical commentators are fundamentally constrained by this overwhelmingly supportive regulatory context. Although the Human Genome Project's Ethical Legal Social Implications Programme and the UK's most recent government commission, the Human Genetics Commission, emphasize the seriousness with which they view their task, their teeth are blunted by a limited remit that largely focuses on public education and the standardization of gene technologies and services. Meanwhile, commercial genomics expands rapidly. We now go on to discuss these issues in greater depth, beginning with the cultural representation of genetics.

7

Genetics as culture

To understand the way that genetics operates today we need to understand the way our culture presents genetics, and draws on genetics for its symbolism. Genetics is also influenced by culture, which shapes its priorities and ways of understanding disease and behaviour. This requires that we be mindful of the past, sensitive to the continuities and changes in both genetics and popular culture. We need to be aware of the ways in which genetics has always been informed by deep-seated values about disability and behaviour, and has, in turn, shaped the public perception and treatment of disabled people, their families and other marginalized groups such as the poor and ethnic minorities.

In this chapter, we will explore three aspects of genetics and contemporary culture. We will begin by looking at how genetics is portrayed in the media and in popular discourse. We will discuss the tendency towards what Canadian health researcher Abby Lippman has called 'geneticization', where a range of human problems are reduced to genetic variations.[1] This reflects the interests of the media, the commercial companies and charities that fund genetics, and geneticists themselves, as we shall discuss. We will also discuss the effects of this portrayal of genetics in wider society, arguing that it reinforces a sense of individual responsibility for health surveillance, rather than addressing the social causes and social responsibilities for health and welfare. To illustrate these processes we will look at behavioural genetics and evolutionary psychology. But we will also point to some ways in which the dominant messages and their effects are subverted by public scepticism and people's direct experiences of the new molecular medicine.

Cultural representations

The science and practice of genetics is a rich source of cultural symbolism. Even before the discovery of DNA and other transmission mechanisms, there was a prior cultural discourse around genetics. Notions of race, inheritance and family have been central to human cultures for centuries. Our discussion of eugenics in the first half of the book showed these ideas at work, as the new sciences tapped into traditional beliefs and fears about degeneration and racial pollution. The metaphor of the survival of the fittest – coined by the sociologist Herbert Spencer, but strongly associated with the Darwinian evolutionary paradigm – was the justification for various strains of social Darwinism, and was notoriously evoked by Adolf Hitler in *Mein Kampf*.

Many scientists argue that it is now possible to draw a distinction between science and society. They say that their work is value free and neutral, and that the controversies emerge around the abuse of scientific discoveries, not science itself. However, this perspective is strongly refuted by social researchers and cultural analysts. The field of genetics deploys a range of metaphors and analogies to explain the molecular processes and to win support for the science. Genetics is part of culture, not outside culture. For example, the genome is described as the 'Holy Grail', the 'Book of Life' or the 'Code of Codes'. Attempts to explain how the science works draw on metaphors such as 'DNA is like a language' or 'the genome is a library' or 'genetics is a blueprint'. Changes that lead to genetic disease are called 'misprints' or 'spelling mistakes'. All these metaphors are culturally situated, drawing on a mixed set of factors such as the authority of the Bible and the social conventions of language and writing, as well as the more recent public appetite for information technology.

In *The DNA Mystique* Dorothy Nelkin and Susan Lindee suggest that the gene has become a cultural icon in American society: 'In both the language of scientists and the parables of popular culture, the biological structure called DNA has assumed a nearly spiritual importance as a powerful and sacred object through which human life and fate can be explained and understood.'[2] When the media report the search for genes for alcoholism, novelty seeking, obesity or homosexuality, they are fuelling the idea that genes determine not only large areas of disease, but also a range of behaviours. As Nelkin and Lindee argue,

> There are selfish genes, pleasure-seeking genes, violence genes, celebrity genes, gay genes, couch-potato genes, depression genes, genes for genius, genes for saving, and even genes for sinning. These popular images convey a striking picture of the gene as powerful, deterministic, and central to an understanding of both everyday behaviour and the 'secret of life'.[3]

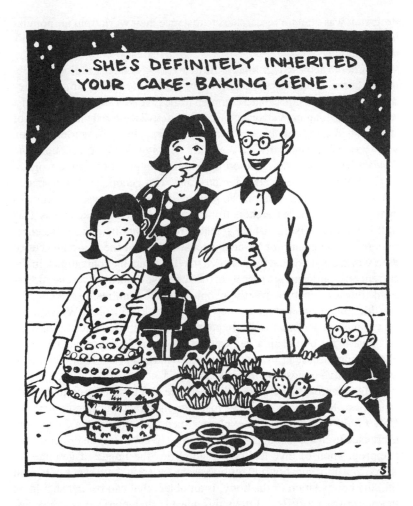

Genetic metaphors have also reached beyond the bounds of health and behaviour. This can be seen in the way that an increasing number of
advertisements draw on genetic or evolutionary connotations. One car
manufacturer even used the British geneticist and media scientist Steve
Jones to promote its new model. The 'gene for' concept has become a metaphor that is used in many areas of life to explain someone's supposed
innate ability, even when no biological connection is remotely suggested.
As Jose Van Dijck notes in her book *Imagenations*, grandiose metaphors
such as these were developed to win public support, and government funding, for genetic big science, in the form of the $3 billion Human Genome

Project. It was vital for researchers to distance their work from the popular images of genetic engineering, environmental risk and Frankenstein's manipulations.

In order to achieve legitimacy, the new biology had to develop the alibi of health and social improvement as the potential benefits of genetic research. Van Dijck notes that a common trope revolves around the scientist as hero. Since James Watson and Francis Crick discovered the structure of DNA, the idea of geneticists as intrepid explorers in a new world has been very powerful, especially in Watson's self-aggrandizing account, *The Double Helix*. Of course, these images pre-date genetics, as the work of H. G. Wells and Jules Verne demonstrates. But geneticists had a special interest in this representation. To legitimate genetics, it was important to distinguish humane researchers from irresponsible Dr Frankensteins. Part of this involved distinguishing science from the applications of science: researchers often call for 'ethical discussion' about the consequences of their work, but deny that the research itself is ethically contentious. In the current era, clinicians are seen as heroes because their work rescues others from illness or enables infertile people to make families. In the UK, the considerable media profile of the IVF pioneer Lord Robert Winston fits Van Dijck's description well: 'In popular stories, the geneticist is primarily staged as a clinician, a dedicated doctor who is not only capable of eliminating disease at its roots, but is also skilled at overcoming ethical and legislative opposition to gene therapy.'[4]

If the scientist is a hero, then the narrative plot is based around the idea of a quest. References are often made to an archetypal quest story, the Holy Grail. Real-life global explorers such as Columbus or Lewis and Clarke are used to illustrate the nature of the Human Genome Project: 'The reappropriation of mythical quests amplifies the image of genome research as a holy vocation and reinforces the idea that the essence of human life, the composition of the body, is an object that can be and should be thoroughly demystified.'[5] Often, this quest is characterized as a race. For example, in Watson's *The Double Helix*, a sense of urgency is rather spuriously provided by the supposed competition with the research team led by Linus Pauling to identify the structure of DNA. The same book also draws on the classic detective story plot, according to Van Dijck. James Watson himself plays the role of the great detective, while the obstacle or villain is provided by the crystallographer, Rosalind Franklin: her work, which was vital to the discovery, is downplayed. The victors write history.

Leading scientists and doctors can appear to be overtaken by the sense of mastery that this portrayal of the drama of genetics evokes when they make dangerous social pronouncements about eugenic improvement. For example, Watson said in 1997:

> We must not fall into the absurd trap of being against everything Hitler was for. It was in no way evil for Hitler to regard mental disease as a scourge on society . . . Because of Hitler's use of the term Master Race, we should not feel the need to say that we never want to use genetics to make humans more capable than they are today.[6]

As we have already discussed, before Watson, the American geneticist H. J. Muller had suggested in 1959 that infertility provides an 'excellent opportunity of making a breakthrough for positive eugenics'. Francis Crick, co-discoverer of DNA, suggested in the 1960s that prospective parents should require a licence in order to reproduce. Although they would undoubtedly blanche at these extreme views, very many doctors and researchers have heralded the benefits of genetic research to health, by which they mean the potential to terminate pregnancy selectively to avoid disabled children. Some experts have developed cost–benefit arguments to show the money that could be saved by the prevention of the births of Down's-affected babies. As Alan Ryan argues, 'Contemporary scientists sometimes seem oddly blind to the fact that other people do not share the rather simple utilitarian vision that they themselves accept.'[7]

The narrative of improving health is mainly on the basis of removing disabled people from the world, yet scientists are often ignorant about the experiences and views of disabled people, and seem to ignore the trauma of abortion for pregnant women and their families. Having said that, it would be wrong to single out scientists as apart from culture. Their views may sometimes be expressed with an unpleasantly cold precision, but many people in society at large share their prejudices and fears about disability. It is therefore unhelpful to demonize scientists and clinicians, as environmental activists, radical feminists and the disability movement have sometimes done, by painting geneticists as power-crazed conspirators or even Nazis, and describing genetics as an extermination programme.

Wider cultural attitudes about the tragedy of disability clearly add to the hype about the benefits of the new genetics. But they also impact on the practice of genetics, determining geneticists' priorities. For example, if people with Down's syndrome were not stigmatized and were just considered to be different, there might not have been so much time and money spent on identifying the causes of the disorder and developing better screening technologies to eliminate Down's foetuses. As Van Dijck notes: 'The public appeal of genetics is contingent on the shifting mobilization of images, but also on the projection of imaginations onto theories, practices, instruments or applications of genetics.'[8] Social processes within science reinforce geneticisation too: it is not simply a feature of the presentation of genetics in the media, but the actual practice of genetic research. As Joan Fujimura's work suggests, genetics has become an important bandwagon in medical and scientific research.[9] Researchers looking for money to investigate a particular disorder or trait tend to frame grant proposals around questions of genetics. Let's not forget that these priorities are not entirely altruistic. There is big money in genetic research, and scientists themselves have a lot to gain from setting up companies and obtaining patents, as well as working for large, wealthy pharmaceutical companies.

Geneticization comes from science itself, not just media misunderstanding and sensationalism, as is commonly claimed. By talking up their research, by promising magic bullets and by getting positive media coverage, scientists ensure that corporate shares prosper and more funding becomes available from government or private investors. For example, Van Dijck has demonstrated how the burgeoning in vitro fertilization (IVF) industry was bolstered by the framing of infertility as a terrible plague, and the images of 'desperate' infertile women who needed help. Subsequently, IVF was marketed as the humane solution to this need, and naturalized as a 'blessed technology'. Within this discourse, the spurious idea of an 'epidemic of infertility' was constructed and reproduced in media and medical publications, in order to demonstrate the demand for an 'unproblematic, transparent solution to an opaque, complex medical problem'.[10]

As we have already discussed, Paul Martin has also shown that the reconceptualization of particular diseases (cancers, heart disease, Alzheimer's) as genetic expanded the potential for gene therapy. Whereas in the early stages of gene therapy, pharmaceutical companies were uninvolved – partly because the potential therapies were relevant only to obscure conditions affecting few patients – once common diseases were redescribed in terms of genetic pathology, so commerce became interested. By 1996 over $1 billion had been invested in small gene therapy firms by the pharmaceutical industry in the pursuit of gene transfer drugs.

The debate over legislation on embryo research discussed by Michael Mulkay also illustrates this redefinition process well. He demonstrates how anti-abortion opposition to research was neutralized and sidelined by very positive media representations, based on uncritical acceptance of medical viewpoints:

> Embryo research is justified in articles of this kind by means of an evocation of a better future which will be experienced, not just by a few fortunate individuals, but by anyone who wishes to take advantage of these new reproductive technologies. In the world constructed in these texts, relief from suffering and an increase in joy and happiness follow unproblematically from the advance of scientific knowledge.[11]

A group called 'Progress' was founded by scientists and doctors involved in this research to shape public perceptions of reproductive and genetic technology, and as the Progress Educational Trust it continues to put a positive spin on the latest scientific advances and to argue that regulation is unnecessary or should be reduced.

Rather than seeing scientists as neutral, we argue that they have to be seen as part of society, as gatekeepers who regulate the flow of information to selected journalists and hence to the public. Barbara Katz Rothman points to the role of scientists and doctors in influencing public opinion: they produce culture themselves, sometimes explicitly in the form of books, articles and television programmes, rather than being detached observers. Abby Lippman sees biomedical experts as storytellers – like novelists, shaping material to tell a story – making genetic complexity into an accessible narrative.[12]

Alongside entrepreneurial scientists, keen to boost their profile and deflate restrictive legislation, the media undoubtedly play an important role in legitimating and popularizing genetic science and reductionist explanations. The recent discoveries of genes associated with physical conditions – such as Huntington's disease, dwarfism, muscular dystrophy, cystic fibrosis, breast and colon cancer – have fuelled a willingness amongst journalists to attribute all sorts of behaviours and attributes to the influence of genes. In the 1990s, 'gene for' stories were extremely common. Headlines have reported 'genes for' homosexuality, novelty seeking, bed-wetting, alcoholism and obesity, as well as a whole range of other social experiences. Journalists also use an inaccurate form of shorthand, talking about 'the gay gene' or 'the breast cancer gene' as if there was such a thing, as if there was only one genetic cause, and as if having the gene meant invariably being gay or having breast cancer. American sociologist Peter Conrad has shown how news tends to adopt a frame of 'genetic optimism' and not to report ensuing disconfirmations. Conrad argues that this reflects the logic of news: finding something new is news, but a failure to find it is not.[13]

A good example of this kind of geneticization is provided by Henderson and Kitzinger, who explored the ways in which breast cancer was reported in the media, and found that genetics or inheritance was the main topic of one-third of articles focusing on breast cancer risk, as well as being mentioned in passing in many other stories.[14] However, less than 15% of breast cancers are attributable to the influence of the BRCA-1 and BRCA-2 genes. The genetic stories on breast cancer went beyond simple news coverage, including features, opinion pieces and personal accounts. The latter tended to focus on the dilemmas around testing and prophylactic mastectomy in families affected by inherited breast cancer. Henderson and Kitzinger found that genetic stories on breast cancer had permeated a wide range of media coverage, and were seen as having great value as 'soft' (i.e. human interest) news items: this was because breast cancer genetics touches on powerful media themes such as death, sex, motherhood, choice, secrecy, bereavement and tragedy. Organizations and affected individuals felt that such coverage exaggerated the dramatic and tragic elements of the condition, as well as inflating the role of inherited factors.

The effects of geneticization

So far we have shown that there are a range of groups with an interest in over-emphasizing the importance of genetics. This makes genes seem too central to the human experience. Over-inflated genetic metaphors, such as James Watson's comment that 'we used to think our fates were written in the stars. Now we know, in large part, they are written in the genes', are highly reductionist. The computer metaphor implies that we are passive agents of our DNA programme, like Richard Dawkins' description of human beings as robots for reproducing genes. Calling the genome the Book of Life ignores all the other processes that contribute to our experiences, alongside biology. The American sociologist Barbara Katz Rothman takes exception to the blueprint metaphor because it doesn't contain any reference to time and development, which are central to genetics and reproduction: instead she offers the metaphors of DNA as a recipe or even a musical score.[15] The idea of the Human Genome Project as a translation is also inaccurate: molecular biologists have so far succeeded only in transliterating the genome – as if from Cyrillic to Roman letters. They have not managed to read, but only to name the letters.

While this hype undoubtedly fuels the promise of genetics in the public's mind, it also has a direct impact on people's lives. Henderson and Kitzinger's study of genetics and breast cancer found that most focus group respondents estimated that inheritance accounted for over 50 per cent of breast cancer causation, well above the true figure of 10 per cent. If respondents had a relative who had experienced breast cancer, they felt at risk, while if they did not, they felt complacent about risk. Many had vivid memories of specific human interest stories in the media. This is a clear example of the effects of geneticization: many healthy women seeing themselves as potentially at risk. Geneticization may also raise people's expectations about the imminence of a cure, which doctors are frustrated about their inabilities to provide.

Joseph Alper and Jonathan Beckwith further highlight the danger of genetic fatalism, where genes are seen as determining, causing traits that are unchangeable.[16] This takes attention away from the social causes of disease and 'anti-social behaviour', reducing funding for research and support schemes to counter the social situations that foster health inequalities. For example, in the case of type 2 diabetes, it is well known that diet and environment play a crucial role. Yet there has still been a major search for the genetic factor. Rather than trying to alter behaviour or the social context, scientists tend to promote a genetic solution to particular problems, often because genetic solutions can be commodified, generating profit, whereas social change and health promotion are not areas with commercial potential. Another example of this is the case of alcoholism, where a Californian winemaker has funded the Ernest Gallo Clinic and Research Centre at the University of California at San Francisco: finding a genetic cause of alcohol addiction would further medicalize this social problem, removing blame from its commercial producers.

In the field of social policy, reducing complex human problems to genetic defects has a wider political impact. This is most clear in the early twentieth-century articulation of eugenics, where poverty or crime or social dislocation was blamed on problem families or generalized racial degeneration. But, as we have argued throughout this book, these practices are not confined to the distant past. As we have already discussed, in the 1960s, some studies showed a high level of chromosomal abnormalities among the population of criminally insane. It was alleged that there was a twenty-fold increase in the prevalence of the XYY genotype. This led to great media sensation and public interest, and generated serious plans to screen for the condition. Only subsequently was it demonstrated that 96 per cent of XYY males were not criminal at all, and that screening would only increase stigma and discrimination. Recently, as we discuss more fully in Chapter 9, new ideas about what Nikolas Rose has called 'biocriminality' are impacting on social policy in a way that is likely further to fuel inequality and discrimination.

Geneticization also has implications for social policies beyond those concerned with crime. As Kaplan points out, genetic research into obesity and mood-affective disorders, for example, emphasize individuals' predispositions to 'poor brain chemistry' over their social situations, suggesting targeted pharmaceutical solutions that are the responsibility of the 'patient' to administer, and undermining efforts to change the patient's environment or foster a society that is tolerant of different temperaments and sizes.[17] Of course, it would be foolish not to acknowledge the value of certain drugs in the treatment of the most serious forms of these conditions, or to disregard the difficulties they pose for those affected. But we must caution that the expanding categories of conditions like depression and obesity, and the related emphasis on genes over environments, undermines a more holistic and tolerant approach to difference and distress.

Genetic discourses as well as genetic technologies and treatments can also reinforce existing prejudices. In the USA, there has been a notorious tendency to explain the poor educational attainments and limited socio-economic prospects of inner-city African Americans by a supposed genetic intellectual inferiority, as in Charles Murray and Richard Herrnstein's book *The Bell Curve*. Charles Murray has recently claimed that 'genetics demolishes left wing egalitarianism, by proving that men and women are suited to different social roles ... the population below the poverty line in the US has a configuration of the relevant genetic makeup significantly different from the configuration of the population above the poverty line'.[18] If racial minorities or poor people are doomed because of their biological inadequacy, the state or the ruling classes are relieved of any obligation towards income redistribution or welfare services. If crime is a product of genetics, then the contribution of deprivation and social exclusion need not be analysed or reformed. As Nelkin and Lindee argue: 'The idea of genetic predisposition encourages a passive attitude toward social injustice, an apathy about continuing social problems, and a reason to preserve the status quo.'[19]

It is important to counter this discourse of genetic determinism, not only in the area of social behaviours, but also around the genetics of disease. As we have observed, the language of 'gene for' is highly inaccurate. There are no gay genes or criminal genes. Biologists Patrick Bateson and Paul Martin reiterate this important point: 'no simple correspondence is found between individual genes and particular behaviour patterns or psychological characteristics. Genes store information coding for the amino acid sequences of proteins; that is all. They do not code for parts of the nervous system and they certainly do not code for particular behaviour patterns.'[20] Thus 'gene for' language is too simplistic: all it can mean is that a genetic difference between two groups is associated with a difference in behaviour. However, it is rarely a single gene that is decisive. For example, polygeny is the process by which many genes contribute to one variation. Often, particular combinations of genes have particular effects: the concept of penetrance is used to explain how one gene may be overridden by other genes. Pleiotropy is the process where a single gene may influence different behaviours. Almost always, the environment plays a major role, alongside the combinations of genes. As Bateson and Martin, Steven Rose and many other leading biologists explain, the 'one gene, one disease', or OGOD, language has limited scientific validity.

Media and popular discourse does emphasize an over-simplified version of Mendelian inheritance to explain the common belief that characteristics 'run in families'. Mendelian patterns of inheritance may account for many rare conditions (about 5,000 single-gene defects), but it is not a useful model for common or complex phenomena, which depend on the interaction of many genes with the environment.

However, we should be wary of some geneticists' attempts to pin the blame for this simplification on the media and public ignorance. Many geneticists promote this type of thinking in the overblown rhetoric of popular science and press releases. We should also be cautious about some of geneticists' criticisms of the OGOD rhetoric because this can involve an implicit message that because the bulk of genetics deals with more than one gene it is unproblematic, if only the public could just grasp its complexity. But accounts of multi-gene interactions and environmental modifiers can be equally determinist. Far from there being a balanced approach to nature and nurture, the fact remains that it is genes that are often the focus of study, not the environment. The study of genes is heralded as a way of understanding the environmental aspects of disease and behaviour, with too little attention being paid to the variability and uncertainties in knowledge about diseases and behaviours. The reductionist paradigm dominates molecular biology and associated disciplines of behavioural and psychiatric genetics, even when more than one gene is identified as contributing to the disorder. The recent claims that the identification of 31,000 as opposed to the expected 100,000 genes in the draft human genome would mean the end of genetic determinism are fanciful in the extreme. Multi-gene explanations are still genetic explanations which often tend to imply genetic solutions and downplay the role of the environment in shaping disease and behaviour.

Social Darwinism and behavioural genetics

Social Darwinism and behavioural genetics are good examples of the kinds of process we have been discussing. Behavioural genetics and evolutionary psychology both seek biological explanations for psychological and social phenomena. Evolutionary psychology does not provide evidence of any specific mechanisms for the hypothetical contribution of genetics, and much of the research emanating from behavioural genetics cannot be replicated, casting doubt on its validity. But the new molecular techniques and the draft HGP offer behavioural geneticists in particular the opportunity to enhance their research with empirical evidence that apparently supports their claims.

Behavioural genetics is a relatively new field of study, linking psychology, psychiatry and molecular genetics. The contribution of genetics to mental disorders such as Down's syndrome and fragile X is uncontroversial, but behavioural geneticists extrapolate into other areas of mental health and personality. For example, it is commonly claimed that schizophrenia and depression arise mainly from genetic factors. Some genes have been identified as being involved in these disorders, but these only have a small effect on a small number of patients and the results are difficult to replicate. In the absence of significant genetic data, arguments for a biological basis to behavioural variations often depend on assumptions about heritability. This is a measure of how much of the variation between individuals is attributable to genetic variation, as opposed to environment, nutrition and upbringing. However, it is a problematic concept. As Patrick Bateson and Paul Martin demonstrate, it is dependent on variables such as the particular population of individuals sampled. For example, height is more heritable in a group of exclusively well-nourished people than amongst people drawn from a wider range of environments. The measure also throws up some oddities: for example, the heritability of walking on two legs or having two ears is nil. This is because the usual source of variation is environmental injury. Yet obviously both ears and legs depend on genetics: as Bateson and Martin conclude, 'a low heritability clearly does not mean that development is unaffected by genes'.[21]

The danger of crude measures of heritability is that they suggest that environment plus genetics creates a particular outcome. Yet the two factors always interrelate: 'the effects of a particular set of genes depend critically on the environment in which they are expressed, while the effects of a particular sort of environment depend on the individual's genes'.[22] The attempt to generate either/or arguments in favour of nature or nurture is doomed to failure. Both genetics and environment play a crucial role, and it is dangerous to reduce complex behavioural phenomena to crude 'genes for' language.

But, once again, we must note that behavioural and psychiatric geneticists are often at the forefront of calls for a more sophisticated, balanced approach to nature and nurture. Robert Plomin talks of a pendulum where in the past we were overly concerned by genetics and heredity (the era of mainline eugenics), and as a reaction to this, research swung to the opposite extreme, where environment was inappropriately privileged, in the 1960s and 1970s. He argues that now, with behavioural and psychiatric genetics, we have reached a point of equilibrium where genes and environment are both considered equally. This rhetoric of balance and neutrality has proved popular in press coverage of this kind of research, and has been important in developing a professional image of responsibility and rigour.

But we argue that the research in this area is far from balanced. Genes and heredity tend to be the focus, not environment.

Measures of heritability are usually based on twin studies, which seem to be the main research activity of behavioural geneticists. This whole research process is highly controversial, given its history of fraud. Little wonder then that contemporary twin studies researchers such as Thomas Bouchard have been reluctant to release all the data from their surveys to researchers seeking to challenge their findings. Where identical twins are more alike than non-identical twins, behavioural geneticists assume that the source of similarity must be genetic, given shared environments. They are particularly interested in identical twins that are reared apart – for example, due to adoption. If they show similar traits, then this is supposedly incontrovertible evidence of genetic influences. However, the shared foetal environment of these children and the fact that they are often reared together for the first part of their lives undermines these claims. Furthermore, when twins are reared apart, it is often in very similar homes with adoptive families who are similar to – and sometimes even genetically related to – the birth family. Many of the supposed correlations may also be pure coincidences, yet they remain endlessly fascinating to the popular imagination and are frequently the topic of quirky media reports, whose humour disguises a potent genetic determinism at work.

There also remains a considerable interest in the genetics of IQ amongst psychologists and psychiatrists. Based on the evidence of twin studies, which seem to show a heritability of 'intelligence' of about 50 per cent, researchers such as Robert Plomin claim that there is a single measure of intelligence, 'g', which can be gauged via IQ tests. This is not to suggest that there is one gene for intelligence, but that quantitative trait loci analysis can find the interacting genes that control this feature of personality. However, these claims are highly controversial. Many psychologists and social scientists deny that there is a single quality called intelligence. Moreover, it is difficult to explain how average measures of IQ can have risen so quickly in the period since the Second World War, if it is an innate, genetically determined phenomenon. Steven Jay Gould in *The Mismeasure of Man*, Ken Richardson in *The Making of Intelligence*, and many others, have cast doubt on the whole process of IQ testing, which is heavily culturally dependent. It is therefore not surprising to see researchers recast their interests for public and professional consumption in terms of cognitive disability. Through researching disorders like attention deficit hyperactivity disorder (itself highly controversial because of the proliferation of Ritalin as a means of treating behavioural disorders in school), behavioural geneticists are continuing their work in cognition in the more palatable role of medical doctor, engaged in health research.

As we have mentioned previously, Dean Hamer, a researcher at the American National Institutes of Health, has made the even more controversial claim that homosexuality involves a genetic component. Alerted by the high heritability of male homosexuality found in some twin studies, his team recruited gay men who had other gay male relatives. Looking at their family trees, they hypothesized that a genetic factor in homosexuality was located on the X chromosome, claiming that this explained the fact that maternal uncles and the sons of maternal aunts showed a higher likelihood of being gay. Analysing samples with statistical techniques, they found that a specific marker showed a significant correlation in the gay subjects. Hamer suggested that the gay gene would eventually be found in this Xq28 region. However, this research was carried out on a very small sample of gay men. Further research has failed to confirm the hypothesis. Despite considerable media hype, claims for a genetic basis to homosexuality seem premature. Yet Hamer's rejection of the 'one gene' storyline did nothing to dampen his or his media allies' interest in hyping the significance of these findings. He even went as far as to claim that this would end the persecution of homosexuals. And as Conrad has shown, much less media interest has been directed to the disconfirmation of the findings, so the genetic explanation of homosexuality remains in the public imagination.

A third example of dubious behavioural genetics is the work on sex roles carried out on girls affected by Turner syndrome.[23] Again, this research generated excited media headlines. Because girls with this restricted growth condition have only one X chromosome, which is sometimes inherited from their fathers and sometimes from their mothers, it was suggested by the researchers that their personality differences provided firm evidence of a genetic basis to the differences between men and women in general. There are several problems with this assumption. First, it is a major leap from a sample of 80 disabled women (average age 13) to the entire human population. Second, the social isolation and other difficulties faced by disabled people may have contributed to the personalities of these women with Turner syndrome, who have a very visible impairment and often also have educational difficulties. Third, the claims about personality arose from a questionnaire filled in by parents, which included items such as 'very demanding of people's time', 'difficult to reason with when upset', 'does not respond to commands', all features which may be quite characteristic of 13-year-old children in general, and perhaps particularly children with mild learning difficulties. It may be that further studies produce further data or identify specific genetic factors. Until then, however, we believe that research of this type should be greeted with scepticism and caution.

We should also be cautious about behavioural and psychiatric geneticists' efforts to enhance their research with genetic data. This involves larger samples and brings individuals without symptoms under their gaze in order to identify what Owen and Cardno have called 'indices of genetic risk'.[24] They continue: 'Studies of this kind will require the identification of large epidemiologically based samples together with the collection of relevant environmental data. This could start now with DNA being banked for future use.'[25] This would entail surveillance of populations on a considerable scale, and raises many questions about informed consent to the future uses of genetic data, confidentiality, patenting of genetic material and inappropriate prying into people's past and present, as we discuss in future chapters. Should any genes be identified for these disorders, the prevailing cultural and social conditions would mean that there would be an increasing emphasis on the responsibility of individuals to be tested for these genes and to take mitigating action, typically pharmaceutical solutions. The current emphasis on a continuum of risk factors is particularly worrying as it brings a large section of the population under the medical gaze, despite their lack of symptoms. This has implications not only for their sense of health and responsibility, but also for their duty as a potential parent, raising the spectre of yet more genetic diagnosis and intervention in conception and pregnancy.

While behavioural genetics seeks evidence for the genetic factors in personality, evolutionary psychology develops hypotheses that attempt to explain contemporary human behaviours and social arrangements in terms of the evolutionary pressures on Stone Age men and women. This descends from the line of argument developed by Richard Dawkins in his 1976 classic *The Selfish Gene*, and it applies biological principles to the human species, just as E. O. Wilson and other 1970s sociobiologists extrapolated from the behaviour of various insects, birds and mammals in order to 'explain' human society. We know that social Darwinism of the early part of the twentieth century included left-wing and right-wing variants, so it would be wrong to assume that evolutionary psychology is invariably associated with conservative ideas about people and society. This is equally true today. For example, the utilitarian bioethicist Peter Singer, a supporter of evolutionary psychology, has argued in favour of a 'Darwin for the left' and the sociologist Helena Cronin has 'reclaimed biology for feminism' in the socialist magazine *Red Pepper*. Together with her LSE-based colleagues she also wrote a report for Demos, the centre-left think-tank, promoting Darwinian approaches.

John Tooby and Leda Cosmides, who have the status of founders of evolutionary psychology, have repeatedly poured scorn on what they call 'the standard social scientific model'. Their project is to reduce all of culture to psychology, and to explain all psychology in terms of Darwinian adaptation in the Stone Age period. They challenge social scientific arguments about the diversity and malleability of social structure and social behaviour, replacing this socio-historical account with the claim that human nature is fixed and universal. Evolutionary psychologists consequently maintain that a whole range of social processes – gender differences, child abuse by step-fathers, age difference in marriage, infanticide – are founded in selective pressures.

The main problem with the evolutionary psychology approach is that it can be extended to explain anything. The technique of 'reverse engineering', where writers in this field take a contemporary human behaviour and hypothesize what Stone Age function this behaviour could have had, can be applied to a vast array of topics. However, both scientists and social scientists have undermined all the key claims of evolutionary psychology. Biologists Steven Rose and Gabriel Dover have criticized the 'bean bag' conception of genetics which underlies the work of Dawkins and his followers: evolutionary psychology claims that there is a correspondence between particular genes and particular behaviours, for which there is no evidence. Neuroscience researchers have shown that the brain is not the fixed, functionally adapted 'Swiss army knife' that Pinker and others claim, developing instead an account that highlights the dynamic role of development and flexibility. Evolutionary theorists have criticized the exclusive focus on adaptation and the failure to understand the complexities of natural selection. Social scientists have shown that there is more diversity to human society and human behaviour than a fixed notion of human nature would allow.[26]

But evolutionary psychology has a powerful appeal. While Tooby and Cosmides are hardly household names, their followers such as Steven Pinker (*How the Mind Works*) and Matt Ridley (*The Red Queen, The Origins of Virtue*) led the bestseller lists during the 1990s. Partly this is because, like Richard Dawkins himself, these authors have a flair for well-written, accessible and interesting narratives. But it is also because they provide simple accounts that reinforce many people's assumptions about the world. Social scientists have made life easier for evolutionary psychology, having virtually abandoned writing popular texts about society and behaviour. In the 1980s and 1990s, social and cultural theory became extremely theoretical and abstruse, retreating into post-structuralist and post-modern discussions that often focused on texts rather than providing insights into everyday experiences and behaviours. Into this gap came writers such as Pinker, Ridley, Robert Wright (*The Moral Animal*) and Geoffrey Miller (*The Mating Mind*). Their explanations, focusing on individuals and biology rather than structures and socio-economics, were in tune with a world dominated by neoliberal politics and a new individualism. Moreover, the success of evolutionary psychology may derive from the reassurance it provides, based on the appearance of scientific evidence. When people are looking for something to believe, but have abandoned both traditional religion and the hope of political progress, the simple claims of Darwinian social theory combine the appeal of the *Just-So Stories* with the metaphysics of faith.

It would, of course, be wrong to discount the role of biology in society. Humans have been shaped by evolution, and there are basic behaviours that arise from selective pressures. However, this is a far cry from suggesting that men and women were 'hard wired' in the Stone Age. Unlike other animals, humans have developed highly complex cultures, based on our capacity to learn and to innovate, and the ability to communicate within generations and between generations through speech and writing. Ensuing social development has taken human societies far beyond the basic instinctual drives postulated by Darwinian theorists, and enabled men and women to exercise choice, to create meaning and to behave in ways that are often counter-selective: for example, by becoming religious celibates, by becoming homosexual, by engaging in risky behaviours, by committing suicide.

Similarly, disorders such as schizophrenia and depression clearly operate at the level of the brain, yet this is not the same as saying that they are determined by genetics. While intellectual impairments often arise from genetic differences, this is not the same as saying that intelligence is a single cognitive ability that derives mainly from genetic factors. Our point here is not that genes do not exist, or that biology does not shape behaviour or disease, but that we cannot interpret the biological influences on behaviour, or for that matter disease, from an Archimedian point of view, divorced from the social world in which we exist. The ways in which we classify disorders and diseases are shaped by culture: the culture of science and medicine, as well as the wider culture of which scientists and doctors are also a part. In many ways, these contemporary cultures favour genetic over sociological explanations. As we have argued, these stories tap into deep-seated notions of heredity and biological foundationalism, as well as reflecting the genetics bandwagon – a powerful technological imperative within science and medicine.

Conclusion

Cultural representations are vital to legitimating the new fields of reproductive and genetic technologies, and to achieving funding and regulatory freedom. Genetic explanations of behaviour and disease are promoted by a range of interest groups including scientists and doctors, funding bodies, the government, the media and the commercial sector. This is a form of hype as well as a form of practice, affecting what gets researched, how the research gets conducted and what tests and treatments are taken up in the wider health service. It affects the practice of scientific research and has an effect on social policies, tending to intensify rather than alleviate discrimination and inequality. But there are a number of reasons for cautious optimism about resistance and subversion of this hegemony.

We must take note of the growing public scepticism about the claims made by geneticists and the popular media about the power of the gene. While recognizing the importance of cultural discourses in shaping public and parliamentary opinion, and the corresponding influence of legal and political debates on popular understanding, there is a danger of assuming that media audiences are passive receptors of cultural messages. Some critics have raised the question of how audiences receive cultural messages about genetics, and whether the Nelkin and Lindee thesis may be overstated. Condit argues that media representations are not as deterministic or discriminatory as Nelkin and Lindee imply from their research. In a study of 137 undergraduate students, Condit found that only a minority held a deterministic interpretation of the blueprint metaphor: most saw genetics as probabilistic, open, partial and malleable. Encouragingly, respondents did not see disability as wholly undesirable, or disabled people as having a bad quality of life.[27] Although we must recognize the limited scope of this study, we should also see it as a cue for further audience research that recognizes the ways in which dominant cultural messages such as geneticization are reinterpreted and sometimes radically undermined by the public.

We should also recognize that it is both patronizing and simplistic to claim that the public are inevitably ignorant or irrational when it comes to genetics. Research by Anne and her colleagues at the University of Edinburgh has shown that the public are capable of sophisticated responses to the challenge of genetics. People have a variety of experiences of family, health care and education which can lead them to challenge simplistic genetic stories and overblown claims about genetic treatments and cures. They are also increasingly sceptical about the commercial–state nexus at the heart of genetic research, and highly critical of patenting, and access to genetic information by insurance companies.[28] As we go on to discuss in Chapter 10, while we must be wary of the industry of pollsters that has emerged in recent years, and about the lack of true public consultation that this can mask, there is ample reason to argue that the public are sophisticated enough to become more involved in policy making about genetics, and that this could even foster a less determinist approach to health and behaviour.

Genetic determinism can also be subverted when it impacts on individuals affected by genetic disease in their families. As Novas and Rose have shown in relation to Huntington's disease, people interpret their condition in a variety of ways.[29] Their understanding of genetics cannot be set apart from their other attitudes about health, life and family. Some even choose not to know their disease status, as we discuss further in the following chapter.

We should also note that genetic messages coexist alongside other rhetoric and notions in popular culture, where environment and nurture still play an important role. The hostility in the media and public polls to research into the genetics of intelligence is one example of how genetic messages are not always given carte blanche. Critics of genetic technologies also have a place in some media coverage, especially the traditional debate format. And there are geneticists who are very critical of some research in fields such as behavioural genetics, who sometimes express their reservations in public.

In order to foster these alternative discourses and understandings, and thereby undermine geneticization, we require a variety of approaches. José Van Dijck favours an array of cultural strategies for raising awareness and generating debate, particularly in order to bring marginalized groups into the discussion. The aim of these cultural activities should not be to make them choose or decide, but to make them think. For example, Tom co-ordinates the Policy, Ethics and the Life Sciences (PEALS) project at the Centre for Life, University of Newcastle, which has a writer in residence and has developed visual art activities to enable people of different ages to think about the new genetic and reproductive technologies, and to consider the impact they may have on society. Arts approaches suggest that scientific data are not the only valid form of knowledge. Social scientific research on the attitudes and experiences of participants in new technologies also tells important stories of the practical application of genetics. The personal accounts of disabled people, of women and of children are also important to the development of a more balanced view of the opportunities and threats presented by these new sciences. We discuss these ideas further in the chapters that follow.

8
Choice in social context

Democracies are built on the assumption that people's free choice is the basis of legitimacy. Increasingly, it is consumer choices rather than electoral ones that define identity. Possessions, lifestyle and leisure activities say more about who you are than traditional factors such as employment, politics or religion. In the UK, Margaret Thatcher's policies were built on the notion of free individuals competing in the market place, and able to decide for themselves how to live their lives. The governments that have followed have maintained this emphasis on individual choice. As a result, the UK has become closer to the American ideal of competitive individualism, and choice has been enshrined as a central ethic.

Sceptical commentators would argue that the concept of choice is more of an ideology than a reality. We already know from our discussion of eugenics, in the UK, the USA and Scandinavian countries that democracies do not necessarily involve free choices, particularly about reproductive behaviour. Although eugenics was often presented in the form of voluntary sterilization, there is little doubt that people were coerced. And we must remember that overt coercion remained a feature of eugenics practice even in the 'free world'. Although our experiences today are less overtly constrained by the state, most people, most of the time, have only limited scope for exercising autonomy. After all, if you do not have money, you cannot benefit from a free market. In the UK and the USA, liberalization has been accompanied by an increase in social inequality and relative poverty. The reality of social limitations – the way society structures opportunities – is an important counterbalance to choice. These constraints also operate in the area of healthcare, and particularly genetics. One of the arguments of this book is that the notion of patient autonomy, while benign in theory, masks problems in practice. Individuals do not make their choices in a vacuum, but are influenced by the values and attitudes of society. Medical professionals, families and friends, and the wider public will contribute to the views that patients hold and the decisions they make. But even the notion of choice may be problematic: how far should choice be exercised? What are the ethical limits to individual reproductive autonomy? Who should decide?

The notion of 'informed choice' raises questions about information as well as choice. Genetics has provided new forms of complex information, which can be difficult to interpret. As we have argued, the gene has become a powerful image in contemporary culture. In the past, critics worried about medicalization, whereby complex social experiences are reduced to individual biological pathologies. Now concerns surround geneticization, where genes are seen as the key to human identity and to physical and social problems. For this reason, information provided by genetic analysis has a dangerous status. It may displace the knowledge of pregnant women, mothers and fathers, and people who live with illnesses and impairments. People are experts in their own lives, and their knowledge has to be valued alongside the evidence of genetics and the clinical opinion of doctors.

This chapter explores the choices surrounding the increasing availability of genetic testing. We have already discussed how scientific knowledge of genetics developed during the 1970s and 1980s, and took a massive leap forward in the 1990s with the Human Genome Project, which published the first draft of the genome in February 2001. At the same time, a range of antenatal screening techniques, such as ultrasound examination, chorionic villus sampling, blood serum screening and amniocentesis have been introduced or developed. We now have the capacity to know more than ever before about our genetic characteristics, or the genetic characteristics of the foetus during pregnancy:

> The technical ability to predict a person's future state of health on the basis of present genetic markers creates two new needs: it urges people to find out about their own future chances for a healthy life and procreation, and it raises hopes that the very technology used to determine the causes for defects will also lead to cures.[1]

But knowledge is not necessarily empowering, especially when nothing can be done to alleviate or cure the condition being tested. Either way, the person who is tested bears a heavy burden of responsibility for their or their offspring's future health or behaviour. The new genetic knowledge raises new dilemmas. How should people take advantage of the power of genetics in their own lives? How should they let genetic information influence their reproductive choices? Who else might gain access to this knowledge and use it to discriminate against people with genetic conditions? What's the point of knowledge about future illnesses if nothing can be done to treat them? Can people understand and cope with genetic risk?

The contemporary capacity for knowledge of genetic or developmental disorders has outstripped our ability to cure or ameliorate such conditions. When a pregnancy or a person is tested for particular genetic conditions, either because a family has an increased likelihood of that condition or because of a screening programme, there is a limited range of options for action. At the current time, there are many genetic conditions for which there are no treatments, or few effective treatments. The much heralded benefits of gene therapy are nowhere to be seen, and will not help most impaired people for decades or generations to come.

Sometimes, knowledge of genetic predispositions may help individuals avoid harmful behaviours or environments. For example, someone found to have alpha-antitrypsin deficiency, which increases sensitivity to pollution, would be ill-advised to smoke or to work in certain industries. Someone found to have an inherited risk of breast cancer can have regular check-ups to detect tumours early, or may make the decision to have a mastectomy. Even here, increased anxiety may be the main outcome of knowledge, because screening or even mastectomy may have limited effect. However, the most controversial issues arise where the information obtained relates to a foetus, when there is an option of selective termination of pregnancy.

What are the aims of reproductive screening programmes?

There seems to be confusion or even obfuscation about the reason for the massive investment in reproductive screening programmes. Whereas in the past, the medical profession was more open about the intention of avoiding the birth of affected children, the desire to avoid comparisons with eugenic abuse and the dominant ethic of autonomy have led to equivocation about the purpose of screening, both at the clinical level and in policy terms.

The widespread take-up of prenatal ultrasound is an example of this.[2] Ultrasound is a technology of surveillance. The drive to scan almost all pregnancies does not have as its primary motivation the desire to provide pretty print-outs for expectant mums. It is justified in cost–benefit terms, as one of the main methods of detecting foetal abnormality and preventing the birth of babies with genetic or developmental defects. Whereas ultrasound has become part of many people's positive experience of pregnancy, in a small proportion of cases ultrasound is the precursor to termination of pregnancy. This hidden role of ultrasound is rarely explicitly acknowledged.

This may be because of an unwillingness to raise anxiety. After all, only a tiny proportion – a few per cent – of pregnant women receiving scans will turn out to have an affected foetus. But it might also be the case that if pre-scan information were more direct and explicit, many couples might choose not to have access to that diagnostic power.

Angus Clarke argues that there is a complex relationship between the stated goals of a genetic screening programme, its ethos, and the outcome measures that are used to evaluate it.[3] He suggests that there are three possible goals of screening: avoiding costly disorders; avoiding the suffering of affected children; and promoting informed reproductive decisions. Within the context of public health economics, any screening programme is justified in terms of the benefits derived versus the costs incurred. Prenatal screening programmes are introduced when an argument can be made that the total cost of screening the relevant population is less than the medical and welfare costs of the ill or impaired babies who would otherwise be born. We believe that these equations are immoral when applied to reproductive decision making. They serve to increase prejudice against disabled or different people, and to increase pressure on women to terminate affected pregnancies. There are distinct echoes of the past in these types of cost–benefit analysis, where the social cost of disabled people was used as a reason to sterilize and even murder children and adults. Now we have a more efficient and early method of termination, but this does not make screening moral. As Clarke argues, why should prenatal screening be the only part of the health service that has to make a profit? We agree with his judgement that this approach is dangerously eugenic.

Consumer demand and the rights of prospective parents to make informed choices about their pregnancies are also used to justify screening programmes. Yet the reality is that people's options and choices are far from value free. As Clarke argues, and as we will demonstrate below, the ethos of screening and obstetric services can undermine the possibility of informed consent and just outcomes. This is particularly apparent in the trend towards routinization of testing and the assumption that termination of pregnancy is the inevitable response to a diagnosis of disorder. Once screening programmes are up and running they become entrenched in the health care system. This makes them difficult to challenge for clients and critics alike. It also means that it is far easier to 'bolt on' more and more tests to each screen, because the screening infrastructure as well as the screening culture is well established. The assumption of termination within this culture is starkly illustrated when we consider the different reactions amongst health care providers and society at large to different consumer demands. If a prospective parent wants to select a foetus on the grounds of sex, this is viewed as unethical. If a disabled person wants to select in order to have a child with their own condition – such as deafness – this is also viewed as unethical. In other words, professionals will support consumer choice, as long it is a consumer choice that they think is sensible and ethical. To many disabled commentators, this suggests a double standard. It also suggests that the underlying motivations for genetic screening programmes are not the provision of choice at all, but rather a eugenic aim to avoid the birth of disabled children.

Presymptomatic screening of children or adults apparently avoids many of these eugenic connotations, based as it is on providing people with information so that they can manage their lifestyle or health more effectively in order to prevent or delay the onset of symptoms. For example, genetic screening for colorectal cancer can identify a predisposition to the disease and that an individual can then engage in regular colonoscopies to detect early signs of cancer. Similarly, women with a risk of hereditary breast or ovarian cancer might engage in more regular mammographies or even prophylactic hysterectomy or mastectomy. But these kinds of screening programme are not as benign as they might at first appear. Genetic information is powerful because it has implications for other family members, as well as insurance and employment, as we go on to discuss in the next chapter. Presymptomatic testing can also have implications for reproductive behaviour, as in the case of Huntington's disease, where anecdotal evidence suggests that people are being offered antenatal diagnosis only on the basis that they will abort the foetus if it is found to have the disease gene, despite the fact that Huntington's is a 'late onset' disease, which means that a person can live well into their forties or fifties without any symptoms. As more presymptomatic tests are developed, a 'side-line' in reproductive testing also emerges, and with it many of the problems of antenatal screening.

We should also note that restrictions on choice and eugenic outcomes are not solely confined to antenatal screening services (although this is undoubtedly where they become most problematic). As we said earlier, genetic information is familial information. This can mean that other family members themselves pressurize their relatives into being tested. Choices are further restricted in similar ways to the restrictions on prenatal screening, in terms of the amount and quality of information, and the attitudes of the doctors and nurses. This might mean that people engage in presymptomatic testing even when the benefits of this are far from clear: further health surveillance, prophylactic surgery and lifestyle management may simply increase anxiety and are far from a guarantee of a life without illness. Even the genetic disease they are intended to prevent can still reappear, as in the cases of some women who have had their breasts removed and have subsequently developed ovarian cancer.

For these reasons, we are cautious about the introduction of further genetic screening programmes. Genetic testing in families with a history of a particular condition is less problematic: families will have more knowledge of the condition, and there is more scope for counselling. But as these tests expand, problems of information and service provision come with them. Screening of entire populations is particularly problematic when it becomes a fishing expedition, in which a whole range of conditions may be detected in the pregnancies of couples, who may be given biased and inaccurate information about the impairment concerned. Routinization of prenatal services may further undermine the possibility of informed consent. We therefore favour restriction of further genetic screening and a careful review of existing services.

A common challenge to this kind of position is the argument that people should have the right to screening programmes, wherever they live: in other words, that there should be equity of provision. The Institute for Public Policy Research recently made this case, and the British Medical Association has expressed concern that insufficient screening services and unfair access could lead to the creation of a genetic underclass: middle-class people might take advantage of genetics to have healthier babies, while disadvantaged groups continued to have children with illnesses or impairments. While we recognize the dangers of a two-tier system of screening, especially within the current trend towards the covert privatization of health care, this is not a reason to provide inadequate and prescriptive services through the National Health Service. We can also point out, while inequalities in wealth and opportunities can mean that middle-class people are more likely to take up screening services, they can also mean that they have more resources to raise a disabled child. What is required to promote equality is a careful review of existing screening and health and welfare services for people affected by genetic disorders, for the two cannot be divorced.

Are people able to make informed choices?

The aims and structures of genetic screening and genetic testing clearly influence people's decisions to go ahead with testing. This results in three main factors that significantly undermine people's abilities to make free and informed choices about genetic testing and screening: the information that they are given; the attitudes of medical staff; and the routinization of prenatal services.

First, in order to exercise a real choice, full information about the diagnosis and prognosis of a genetic or developmental condition is vital. But this is lacking in a number of regards. For example, genetic diseases might be caricatured as 'terrible conditions'. One research project found that prospective parents were given an overly pessimistic explanation of the effects of cystic fibrosis.[4] They were given estimates of life expectancy that were much lower than those already being achieved. The range of severity of genetic conditions or the different types of symptom might also not be explained to all parents. Different parents get given different information. Research found that parents whose babies were found to be affected by Down's syndrome were given a much more positive prognosis than those who were being offered a prenatal test and the possibility of selective termination.[5] It is also often the case that genetic information cannot predict the severity or range of symptoms of the condition in a particular individual, as we go on to discuss in the next section.

But clinical information is only part of the picture. In order to understand the implications of a prenatal diagnosis, prospective parents need to be informed about the social experience of disabled people. They might want to know whether people with a particular condition have a good quality of life; whether they can go to mainstream schools; what employment options are available; and what the options are for independent living and welfare benefits. All these issues are important in understanding the impact of impairment on the lives of disabled people. For many disabled people, impairment is a fact of life, not a medical tragedy. They have a good quality of life and achieve the same goals as non-disabled people. Many disabled people argue that the main problems they face are caused by society, not their impairments. The solution to disability is removing social barriers and prejudice, not removing disabled people from society. These perspectives suggest that it may be particularly important to listen to the testimony of disabled people themselves, who are the people directly affected. Ruth Bailey, a disabled activist who has researched prenatal screening and reproductive choice, argues:

> Politicians, scientists and doctors alike must recognise that disabled people do have a particular interest in prenatal testing and should therefore be systematically involved in debates about prenatal testing. This would provide some general insights into the complexities of the experience of disability and impairment, and help to correct many of the current misconceptions.[6]

Yet the voice of disabled people is rarely heard in prenatal situations, which are dominated by doctors and nurses.

A lot of people are ignorant about disability. They might not know any disabled people. They may be deeply fearful about disability. They may think it must be the worse thing that could ever happen to someone. But, as we have argued, disabled people usually don't think like this, and have developed a civil rights approach to the disability problem. Yet this social approach is not usually shared by members of the medical profession. They have been trained to think of illness and impairment as a problem that must be solved through medical intervention. If a condition cannot be cured, it is not illogical for them to think that it should be prevented. Yet in the case of congenital impairments, this means removing the person, not just removing the disease.

People facing difficult decisions often want guidance from experts: the responsibility for deciding may be too heavy for them to bear on their own. Yet counselling and support may be unavailable or inadequate. This also affects the quality and quantity of information provided to people contemplating or participating in genetic screening. Jo Green has found that 45 per cent of obstetricians said they had inadequate resources for counselling women about serum screening for Down's syndrome, the commonest form of prenatal testing.[7] For rarer and more complex conditions, information and advice are even more limited. Green's research also found that women were confused about the new tests: 81 per cent of obstetricians in the study claimed that 'women not understanding the test' was a problem. These problems occurred in the past within a limited screening programme. As screening becomes available to more women for more prenatal conditions, then the shortfalls of the resources and services will become more acute.

This brings us on to our second restriction on choice: the attitudes of medical professionals. The idea that doctors and nurses are non-directive is a myth. Non-directiveness is a goal of counselling, but research has found that it is usually not achieved in practice. This varies according to the professional involved. Marteau and colleagues have found that genetic counsellors and nurses are least directive, obstetricians are most directive and geneticists are somewhere between the two. The extent of obstetricians' directiveness is particularly worrying. Unlike genetics professionals, obstetricians do not tend to work with disabled people directly. They are concerned with delivering the 'perfect baby'. They tend to believe that selective termination of pregnancy is a good idea in the case of many impairments. For example, in cases of Down's syndrome, 94 per cent of genetic nurses, 57 per cent of geneticists, but only 32 per cent of obstetricians reported counselling non-directively. The majority favoured termination of foetuses with open spina bifida, anencephaly, Huntington's disease, Down's syndrome and Duchenne muscular dystrophy, and a substantial minority favoured termination of foetuses with cystic fibrosis, sickle cell anaemia, achondroplasia, PKU and haemophilia.[8] Research by

Wendy Farrant in 1985 found evidence for eugenic beliefs amongst obstetricians, for example the belief that genetic testing is a good thing because it allows people to have healthy babies instead of unhealthy babies; placing a negative value on people with certain conditions; seeing it as desirable to prevent the births of certain foetuses; and erroneously believing that a genetic predisposition to homosexuality can be identified, and that it might be acceptable to terminate selectively on these grounds.[9] Follow-up research by Jo Green in 1995 found that these attitudes had changed. However, one-third of obstetricians would still not give a woman diagnostic testing unless she agreed to have a termination of pregnancy if the foetus was affected by impairment.[10]

A recent Australian case starkly illustrates the extent of directiveness in some obstetric care. In 2000, the coroner in the state of Victoria ordered an investigation into the case of a 40-year-old woman whose pregnancy was terminated at the Royal Women's Hospital at 32 weeks after she learnt that her baby was likely to be a dwarf. Restricted growth is not a life-threatening condition. In fact, it has relatively minor effects on quality of life, and most people who have restricted growth live happy and fulfilled lives. However, contemporary research by the Murdoch Children's Research Institute found that almost 80 per cent of obstetricians would support termination of pregnancy when the foetus had dwarfism. Support for termination at 13 weeks was unanimous among those obstetricians who are expert in diagnosing dwarfism by ultrasound. Support for aborting foetuses with dwarfism at 24 weeks dropped considerably amongst obstetricians in Victoria, from 78 per cent to 14 per cent. But amongst clinical geneticists and obstetricians around Australia who specialize in ultrasound (the main method by which dwarfism is diagnosed), and who were surveyed separately from the Victorian obstetricians, support for termination at 24 weeks remained high, at more than 70 per cent.[11]

This kind of pressure from professionals involved in people's care does not have to be overtly oppressive for it to have a fundamental impact on how information is presented and how the doctor reacts to their client's decision. As one pregnant disabled woman interviewed by Anne and her colleagues at Edinburgh describes,

> I don't think the test for disability in the unborn child is presented as a choice, when I said I didn't want to be tested the doctor was shocked and she tried to talk me into it because it's an easy test, everybody gets it done nowadays, it's simple. But I don't think there is a choice, I think that we're pressured into taking as many of these tests as are available.[12]

The views that professionals hold are important in shaping people's decisions. The way clinicians present options encourages people to engage in particular behaviours. But doctors are not bad people. In fact, their views probably reflect those of many members of the public: the problem therefore is that doctors and nurses are ordinary people, whereas sometimes we expect them to be wise and enlightened. Doctors are not brainwashing or coercing their clients. There is no evidence for such a crude process of influence. The sociologist Stephen Lukes talks about power being exercised in structural rather than individual ways. This may not involve overt conflict, but may be based in cultural processes and social patterns. The exercise of power may appear to be consensual:

> A may exercise power over B by getting him to do what he does not want to do, but he also exercises power over him by influencing, shaping or determining his very wants. Indeed, is it not the supreme exercise of power to get another or others to have the desires you want them to have?[13]

The exercise of power in the genetics clinic is complex and subtle, but ever present.

The third restriction on choice that we focus upon here is the routinization of screening and testing. Obstetric procedures can be like a conveyor belt, where testing may take place without the knowledge of the pregnant woman, or where testing is presented as a routine procedure. Thousands of women are going through antenatal and obstetric services in the NHS, and time and resources are not allocated to ensure that they are fully informed and consenting freely. The very existence of a test for foetal abnormality can create pressures to use the technology. The implication is that testing and selection are desirable outcomes. Therefore it is naive to say that technology is neutral, because the possibility of obtaining prenatal genetic information inevitably creates new problems and solutions that were not previously available.

Research has also shown that women are not encouraged to exercise control in the antenatal setting, and that they place considerable trust in the expertise of their advisers.[14] In her early study Farrant found that a quarter of consultants said their policy was to give the serum screening test routinely without offering women any explanation of its purpose or any choice about whether or not they participated in the screening programme. Another research project by Marteau and colleagues found that one-third of pregnant women who had been offered serum screening to detect spina bifida could not correctly recall whether they had undergone the test.[15] Down's syndrome screening, the most widespread current programme, has many of these problems. First, women over 35 are offered a serum test. This is a straightforward blood test with no risk. But it is not definitive and only indicates a higher risk. There would seem no reason not to have such a test: after all, it's what everyone else does. Of course, serum screening has associated problems, such as anxiety that persists even after a negative result, and confusion and distress about the meaning of the process, but this does not tend to be discussed when a woman is offered testing. Second, if the test is positive – finding a higher likelihood of a Down's pregnancy – the couple are offered an amniocentesis. This is an invasive test that is associated with a raised risk of miscarriage. However, the only point in having a serum test was to see if an amniocentesis was appropriate. Having had the serum test, it seems an obvious next step to have the amniocentesis. Rayna Rapp reports in her book *Testing Women, Testing the Fetus* that in the USA couples have a one-hour counselling session before making this decision. In the UK, little or no formal counselling is usually available.

In a tiny proportion of cases, and after a considerable wait, the amniocentesis might indicate that the foetus has Down's syndrome. At this stage, the couple have to decide whether to act on this result and abort the foetus. And, as with many similar reproductive choices, they do not have much time to make their decision. They may not have thought as far as this. But in the small choices to have a serum test and then an amniocentesis, they have virtually made the big decision of terminating a pregnancy. The clinical staff will certainly expect this outcome: after all, why take a risky test like amniocentesis unless you are prepared to act on the results? The idea that people may just want to know, but might not want to stop the pregnancy, does not carry much weight in the context of screening services.

Nowhere in this scenario have we suggested that couples are coerced or brainwashed. However, neither are they always explicitly told at the beginning of the process that one outcome is termination of pregnancy: they are not asked to decide upfront what they might do if all the tests are positive. In the UK they are not even given proper counselling where there is time to make a better decision. Perhaps to do so would be to make thousands of women and men anxious, just so that one woman and man can be more prepared for a difficult decision. Yet testing already makes people anxious: the problem is that they have not had the time to think clearly in advance, and so some people find they have to make a difficult decision, under pressure of time, which many of them wish they did not have to take responsibility for. The evidence shows that 90 per cent of couples in this situation terminate the pregnancy affected by Down's syndrome. Of course, most of the 30 per cent of women who say they would not consider termination on grounds of foetal abnormality are unlikely to have gone down this route in the first place. Jo Green and Helen Statham capture this well when they say that the routine use of screening means that

pregnant women do not necessarily make an informed decision to undergo screening and diagnostic tests. They may not see it as appropriate
to make a decision, they may not be given information on which to
make a decision, may not read or understand information they are
given, or may not know they are having a test.[16]

We have outlined three arguments for profound concern about the exercise of reproductive choice in prenatal screening. Some of our concerns also
apply to the expansion of presymptomatic testing and screening. It is important to be clear about our claims. We are not suggesting that people
contemplating genetic testing are denied any choice. We are not suggesting
that they are coerced dupes. However, we are suggesting that inadequacy
of information, the role of doctors and the routinization of the testing context create situations where a free and informed choice may not be
available. A common definition of eugenics is 'a population policy based
on coercion'. The contemporary situation involves a multitude of individual decisions. Yet a *de facto* population policy is developing in some
genetic screening programmes. Where many of these individual decisions
may not be free or fully informed, then we argue there is a major risk of eugenic outcomes. This is all the more worrying when we consider the
cost–benefit justifications of screening, which emphasize the number of
disabled lives prevented and the saving to society of such an action: clearly
eugenic statements. Although professionals advocating screening programmes disavow eugenic intent, and make ritual statements about the
need for choice and autonomy, the effect of the policies and programmes
may be to undermine choice. Once more, this is not to demonize health
care professionals, but to question the structures and assumptions that
inform their practices. There is an urgent need to reform genetic testing
and screening procedures to avoid these problems, and to provide a proper
choice to women and men. We argue that no new screening programmes
should be introduced until these issues have been resolved, and that we urgently need to rethink existing programmes rather than simply carry on as
before.

Uncertainty and risk

In a certain sense we could argue that restrictions on choice are also built
into genetic information in its current form. These restrictions come from
uncertainty. Although genetic knowledge is developing all the time, it
remains incomplete. The interaction of genes and their influence on
development are immensely complex. The simple Mendelian patterns of

inheritance and the straightforward OGOD scenario are of limited explanatory power. The gap between genotype (an individual's genetic make-up) and phenotype (how this translates into anatomy and physiology or symptoms and their severities) may be considerable. This means that genetic tests have inherent flaws and limitations.

Even single-gene conditions are highly complex. For example, in the case of Huntington's disease, 2–3 per cent of at-risk individuals will be in a grey area of uncertainty as to whether they will be affected. There are at least 900 separate mutations that can lead to cystic fibrosis. And there are over 200 mutations in the BRCA genes that predispose to breast cancer, but even with a mutation, the risk of breast cancer may only be 50 per cent. In these situations, causality becomes very complex. Different genes interact to modify each other. Genes interact with the environment all the time. This means that it is often difficult to predict whether a potential person will be affected by a condition, or how severely. Barbara Katz Rothman's discussion of sickle cell anaemia illustrates this well:

> Genetically, this illness is understood about as well as anything has ever been understood. That understanding buys you little in the way of prediction and nothing in the way of treatment. Why is one child in agony and another mildly affected? And what can we do to help the one in pain?[17]

When prospective parents deal with genetic risk, they are dealing with uncertainty about how severely a potential child may be affected. For example, some people with cystic fibrosis die in childhood. Others live into their early forties. That is a significant difference in prognosis, which may well affect the way people regard the condition, and the choices they make prenatally. To take another example, the chromosomal condition Down's syndrome varies considerably in its effects. Some Down's children have severe heart defects. Not all Down's children have the same intellectual limitations: some have limited cognitive or communication abilities, while others may be more able, and some even get GCSE qualifications. These factors may influence reproductive choice, but are hard to diagnose prenatally.

This means that genetic answers are expressed in terms of risks and likelihoods, rather than 'yes' or 'no'. For example, fragile X is the second most common cause of learning difficulties after Down's. Screening is apparently straightforward. The condition primarily affects boys, though one-third of carrier females have some intellectual impairment. But this raises difficult dilemmas for prospective parents in the case of an affected female foetus who may or may not be disabled. On other occasions, anomalies are detected via prenatal screening, but the diagnosis and prognosis are uncertain. For example, ultrasound examination may raise suspicions of an abnormality. The technician may note something unusual. The obstetrician or foetal medicine specialist may be alerted. Further consultations may take place, perhaps subsequent scans. Meanwhile, the prospective parents may be waiting, increasingly anxious, increasingly confused, and often not properly informed. Finally an explanation may arrive, couched in caution and uncertainty, and perhaps conveyed in language that is hard to understand. Is it a visual abnormality or a birth defect? How serious is it? And what should be done?

Most people believe it would be better to get reliable information at an earlier stage, so that termination of pregnancy can be less traumatic, the foetus much less advanced and recognizably baby-like, and the process made easier for all parties. We are sympathetic to this position. Yet the danger is that if termination becomes quicker, easier and earlier, it will become more routine. Barbara Katz Rothman asks: 'With later prenatal testing, the question has been how can a woman bear to end a wanted pregnancy? With earlier testing, we face a new question: how can you bear to continue? How much can you know and still go on?'[18] The current stress and difficulty of late termination is a major obstacle to increasing selection in pregnancy. If termination were easier, it might be used for less serious conditions, and be seen as less problematic. This obviously increases the danger of eugenic outcomes and the tentative pregnancy that Rothman warned about in her research on amniocentesis. She discusses the way that women become pregnant, but do not allow themselves to anticipate birth and motherhood until they have undergone a battery of tests which prove that their child is 'healthy': 'The tentatively pregnant woman has entered the pregnant status, she is a pregnant woman, but she knows that she may not be carrying a baby but a genetic accident, a mistake. The pregnancy may not be leading to a baby but to an abortion.'[19]

We should also note that there are many dilemmas and uncertainties for predictive diagnosis in adults. The benefit of current genetic research into multifactorial conditions is increasing understanding of the mechanics of very common diseases such as diabetes, heart disease, high blood pressure, cancers and Alzheimer's, promising better, more targeted pharmaceuticals. But the complex interactions of genes and environment mean that no definite diagnostic information is available for individual patients, who can only be warned of a hypothetical risk or susceptibility. It is important to point out that this 'predisposition' is not the same as 'prediction': 'People diagnosed as predisposed to a behaviour or disease may find themselves treated as if their fate were certain, even when the relationship between the genetic defects and their manifestation in actual behavior or illness is conditional and poorly understood.'[20] Genes are not determining, but the privileging of genetic information in the laboratory, the clinic and the media is deceptive. Instead genetic testing can often generate more rather than less uncertainty about health and disease.

Is knowledge power, or is ignorance bliss?

Whether genetic testing provides firm knowledge of a positive diagnosis or provides more uncertainty, it might be better, in some circumstances, not to know this information. But genetic testing is proliferating and proper counselling is difficult to sustain. Clearly, the information conveyed in genetic tests can cause considerable stress and anxiety, and raise questions of confidentiality as we shall go on to discuss. In recent years, more pharmaceuticals have become available over the counter, and there has been greater willingness to undertake home diagnostics: for example, home tests for pregnancy, blood pressure and blood cholesterol are available. This raises the prospect of over-the-counter or postal genetic testing. Although the British company that set up cystic fibrosis carrier screening by post has discontinued this service, recently another company called Sciona has set up a confidential screening service for individuals to buy online, targeting genes involved in metabolism, the results of which are combined with results from a lifestyle profile to produce a personal 'action plan' to help them to manage their health and well-being. The company plans to have its testing kits available for purchase over the counter at health clubs, private clinics, chemists and health food shops.

More widespread commercial genetic testing is on the horizon. This raises a range of problems:

- inaccuracy of tests, uncertainty of the results and misinterpretation of the results;
- inadequate counselling and support available;
- the possibility that children might be tested;
- inappropriate use of genetic information by employers or insurance companies.

It would be in the interests of commercial providers to exaggerate the power and significance of the tests in order to increase the market for them, with a consequential risk of mis-selling and bad advice. In 1995 the House of Commons Select Committee on Science and Technology warned: 'There is a very real danger that unscrupulous companies may prey on the public's fear of disease and genetic disorders and offer inappropriate tests, without adequate counselling and even without the lab facilities necessary to ensure that they are conducted accurately.'[21] Negative social consequences might also arise from genetic information because of discrimination in insurance and employment. If an individual is not aware of these possible consequences, they might opt for an NHS test, or a commercial test, only to face problems later when they are asked to disclose results.

But there are also intrinsic downsides of testing, even when it is does not reveal that the individual themselves has a disease or a predisposition to disease. Carrier and pre-symptomatic testing demonstrate how a whole new class of patients – the 'healthy ill' – has been created by the new genetics. For example, people may be tested to find if they are carriers of a recessive genetic condition. Because the details of Mendelian genetics are still not widely understood, it may be difficult for people to grasp the notion of carrier status: research has found that some individuals who are informed that they are carriers later feel themselves to be unhealthy, even though they have no clinical reason to believe this. Moreover, people who are carriers may be stigmatised, as was the case with African Americans diagnosed as carriers of the sickle-cell trait in 1970s USA.

When pre-symptomatic testing is available, people from at-risk families have to decide whether to be tested, and have to deal with the stress of finding out that they have a chance of developing the disease themselves. This knowledge has the power to turn healthy people into diseased people, even though they may have no symptoms. Because they carry a gene that may well express itself in the form of illnesses, people may consider themselves, or they may be considered by others, to be unhealthy.

Even for family members who discover they do not carry the gene, there is considerable stress. Research has found 'survivor guilt' and other psychological trauma in members of families affected by difficult diseases, who find that they themselves are unaffected. Sometimes people may have given up the chance of having relationships or children because of genetic risk: finding out that this sacrifice was for nothing may bring resentment and distress. There may be tensions between family members who have the condition, and those who do not.

Nina Hallowell's research on the psycho-social aspects of breast cancer genetics found that women at risk of breast and ovarian cancer feel constrained because of responsibility to other people to determine their risks and to try and control them.[22] Contemporary health promotion preaches that the individual should take responsibility for their health. But people also feel that they have a responsibility not to pass on risk, and to find out information about risk. Feminists such as Barbara Katz Rothman and Deborah Steinberg argue that women in particular are seen as having responsibility, both in terms of transmitting risk to the next generation and in terms of communicating risk to kin. Women may therefore relinquish their own right not to know.[23] New forms of predictive genetic information raise many problems of privacy and responsibility, for which there is no history of social expectations and conventions.

The onset of Huntington's disease (HD) is inevitable and unavoidable for the vast majority of people who have the gene. This gives them the knowledge that they are going to be affected by a very serious and distressing disorder, and sometimes also the age it is likely to affect them. The researcher Nancy Wexler – whose own family is affected by HD – argues that the condition imposes a burden of anticipation and silent apprehension.[24] Since the gene was cloned in March 1993, far fewer people than anticipated have chosen to discover their HD status: only about 12 per cent of at-risk individuals.[25] It is understandable that some people would not want to know bad news. Some research has suggested that the rate of suicide among families affected by HD is four times the average.[26] Yet a dilemma is posed for those at-risk individuals who want to have children: while they cannot do anything about their own fate, they can avoid having at-risk children. But if the foetus is tested and found to have the gene, this automatically provides knowledge of the at-risk parent's status. The only alternative is exclusion testing, where a foetus is tested to see whether the relevant chromosome comes from the potentially affected parent: the pregnancy can be terminated if this is the case. This implies the termination of many pregnancies that have only a 50 per cent chance of resulting in a child with HD.

Prenatal genetic testing creates difficult dilemmas. Sometimes in these cases ignorance is preferable. The new technologies have made every pregnancy a riskier and more difficult business than before, even though infant and mother mortality rates are at their lowest point in history. Rather than leaving things to God or to fate or to chance or to luck, women and men must now take responsibility for impossible choices. As with the myth of Pandora's box, or Adam and Eve in the Garden of Eden, it may not always be good to find everything out. As Barbara Katz Rothman argues,

> The demands of the information age drive us toward getting all the information, toward taking all the control that we can. Perhaps wisdom lies in not always doing so, in making wise judgements about what information we want, and what information we do not want; which choices we want to make, and which choices are not ours to make.[27]

Not only is termination of pregnancy morally significant, it is also deeply traumatic for many women, often for many years afterwards. This is an important element in the debate over screening and reproductive choice. For many women, the choice they face may be between the trauma and stress of having a child who may experience suffering and difficulty and dependency through impairment, and the trauma and stress of ending a wanted pregnancy. We do not believe that both sides of this argument are given equal weight in many commentaries on the prenatal scenario. The use of termination as an option may be seen as straightforward and unproblematic, when in fact it is a choice involving considerable pain, guilt and suffering for women. This is not an argument against termination of pregnancy. But it is an argument for great care and sensitivity in advancing this as a desirable solution to the problem of disability. As Barbara Katz Rothman argues: 'In choosing between the tragedy of a disabled, defective, damaged, hurt, "in-valid" child, and the tragedy of aborting a wanted pregnancy, a woman becomes responsible for the tragedy of her choice. Whichever "choice" she makes, it is all the worse for having been chosen.'[28]

We have argued that discovery of genetic information can cause problems as well as bringing benefits to some people. We believe that prospective parents have the right not to know about the genetic status of their foetus. We also believe that adults have the right not to know about their predispositions to disease. This suggests that a particular caution needs to apply to genetic testing of children. Sometimes, as in the case of the metabolic disorder called phenylketonuria (PKU), detection postnatally enables the administration of treatments for the disease. But often, there are no benefits from early interventions. Meanwhile, testing in childhood removes the right not to know. It also removes genetic privacy, as family members and others may know the results. It could also increase labelling and stigma. Here we agree with those like Angus Clarke and Dena Davis who argue that children should not be tested until they are old enough to decide for themselves.[29]

Is choice a universal acid?

We have highlighted the main justifications of increasing genetic testing: consumer demand, and the right of individuals to make informed choices about their pregnancies and to know their own genetic susceptibilities. We have argued that in practice these choices may be constrained, the knowledge may be uncertain, and it may often be better to remain ignorant, rather than to have the responsibilities that knowledge brings. In this section of this chapter, we want to consider whether the dominance of choice in genetic ethics is appropriate and desirable, and we will focus on the prenatal scenario, because reproductive choice has raised the greatest moral, religious and political objections.

We need to underline once more that we do not oppose termination of pregnancy. When critics of genetics make arguments about the dangers of eugenics, they are often interpreted as being against access to abortion. The debate over reproductive choice is so polarized that many people stand at one extreme or another: either saying that all abortion is wrong, or saying that women should have the right to choose. Often these extremes depend on whether you believe a foetus is a person with rights, or whether you believe that a woman has unlimited control over her body. Those who hold an intermediate position have a difficult task to account for their position. It is always easier to hold to an absolute or extreme argument.

However, there is no logical requirement to be either totally pro-choice or totally anti-choice. In his important and useful discussion, *Life's Dominion*, the philosopher Ronald Dworkin argues against the notion of 'foetal interests' and believes that termination of pregnancy is not immoral. However, he argues that this does not mean that termination of pregnancy is a morally insignificant act. It involves halting life once it has started, and should not be entered into lightly. Because termination of pregnancy is morally significant and important, it should be chosen only when the alternative would be much worse for the parents or potential child.

Dr Gregor Wolbring, a disability activist, scientist and Thalidomide survivor, has argued that a woman's right to choose whether or not to be pregnant should be supported.[30] That is to say, early termination of pregnancy, in cases where a woman has become pregnant by mistake, or has regretted it, or has perhaps been raped or coerced, should be permitted. However, Wolbring and others distinguish this choice not to be pregnant from the choice of 'which foetus to be pregnant with'. They argue that this second choice is illegitimate. Wolbring believes that any decision based on the characteristics of the foetus is discriminatory and immoral. The characteristics of the foetus should be irrelevant in deciding whether or not to continue with a pregnancy. After all, if you are going to allow termination of pregnancy because of factors such as impairment, they argue, then to be consistent you should allow termination of pregnancy because of gender and sexuality and other consumer preferences. Asch and Geller argue that it is not ethically different to select against girls than to select against foetuses with genetic disorders.[31] Ruth Hubbard has compared impairment with ethnicity, arguing that it would be wrong to eliminate ethnic diversity on the basis that racism can cause problems for black people.[32] Like Asch, Geller and Wolbring, she maintains that oppression is more of a problem than impairment. The implication of these critiques is that either characteristics should be able to be taken into account, allowing full choice, or characteristics should be ignored, and impairment selection should be prohibited.

We believe that this approach to choice falls down for two reasons. First, the choice of whether to be pregnant is not absolutely separate from the choice of which foetus to be pregnant with. For example, consider the hypothetical case of a 16-year-old girl who has become pregnant. She may be wondering whether she can cope as a young single mother, and considering the resources and options available to her: she may be keen to continue studying, and eventually to get a job to support herself and her child. She does not want to continue the pregnancy if it means that her whole life is restricted because of lack of education and life chances. The status of the foetus is relevant here: she may consider that it might be possible to combine looking after a non-disabled baby with study and work. However, she might believe that if the baby were disabled, then the extra care and support such a child would demand would prevent her continuing with her other plans: she knows people would be less able and willing to help look after a disabled baby, and that perhaps it would be harder to find suitable child care. Therefore, in this case the decision is not just whether or not to be pregnant, but revolves partly around what sort of baby she might be pregnant with.

The second counter-argument concerns the equivalence between impairment, gender, ethnicity, sexuality and other personality or behavioural characteristics. We believe that there is some similarity between these characteristics. The social model approach in disability studies shows that the main problems for many disabled people arise from social barriers, discrimination and prejudice. Just as women, ethnic minorities, and lesbians and gay men experience social and economic restrictions, so disabled people face difficulties that are not the consequences of their impairments, but are imposed on them by society. So far, so equivalent.

However, we would argue that in the case of impairment, there are also often physical and mental limitations that are intrinsic to the characteristic. Members of other minorities do not have any intrinsic mental or physical limitations: disabled people, to varying extents, usually do. For example, in the case of impairments such as Tay-Sachs disease, Lesch Nyan syndrome and spinal muscular atrophy type II, babies suffer considerable and distressing symptoms, or may die at an early age. In these extreme cases of impairment, it would seem inhumane not to allow women to have access to this information and to have the right to terminate pregnancy on the basis of the characteristics of the foetus.

Of course, not all impairments are of this order. Some impairments like cleft palate and minor deformities seem comparatively insignificant. We believe that it would be unnecessary or immoral for a person to terminate pregnancies affected by these difficulties, which are largely surmountable. This raises the difficult question of how to prevent selective termination on the grounds of minor impairments, trivial differences or behavioural characteristics. These are scenarios where new technology, freedom of information, autonomy and paternalism come into conflict. Our suggestion here is as follows. New tests capable of disclosing this kind of information should not be developed. However, in some cases this information is evident from existing tests such as ultrasound. In these cases either clinicians should not inform parents – as often happens with disclosure of foetal sex – or policy should explicitly forbid termination on these grounds. These dilemmas will become increasingly difficult in future, with gene-chip technologies allowing earlier and more comprehensive diagnosis. This underlines the need for policy discussion of these technologies prior to their development or implementation. The bioethicist Arthur Caplan has argued that the principle of non-directive counselling may seem fine where there is only testing for a few, serious conditions. But with screening tests available for more conditions, not all of which are serious or negative, there is a need for directiveness to discourage immoral requests for termination. Here Ronald Dworkin's argument that termination is morally significant and weighty, and the evidence that the psychological consequences of termination can cause trauma and long-term stress, should be balanced against the desire of some parents to have a 'perfect baby'.[33]

Restrictions in the quality and amount of information around genetic testing, both prenatally and presymptomatically, also lead us to question the value of many of these tests, particularly where there is a significant degree of uncertainty about symptoms and severities, the perspectives of disabled and sick people are not presented and the value of intervention is unclear. Presymptomatic testing also has many risks in terms of access to insurance and employment, as we shall go on to discuss, and these risks ought to be considered most carefully when planning or providing such services.

This means that there is an urgent need for policy-makers to reconsider the quality of choice and information in current and future genetic testing and screening services. Genetics will increasingly provide us with knowledge about the role of genes of small effect, which may create a raised likelihood of a particular condition, but cannot be said to cause it. Some such genes may even be associated with behaviours like shyness or homosexuality, or differences in the normal range – like intelligence or musical ability. There may be powerful social reasons for some prospective parents to want access to this information. Yet, if we are to have a world that supports diversity and equality, it is equally important to prevent selective termination on the basis of such characteristics. Genetic information does not need to lead to a genetic, and in particular a prenatal, solution. Most often, as in the case of the demand for sex selection, the solution lies in increased social education and anti-discrimination measures.

9

The consequences of choice

Building on the analysis of the previous chapter, here we explore three particular social consequences of genetic choices. First, we discuss the wider social context of prenatal screening. Societal pressures are making it increasingly difficult to have a disabled child. The same factors may lead to the development of 'designer babies' in the foreseeable future. Second, we look at the lack of privacy surrounding genetic knowledge, and the dangers of insurers and employers accessing genetic information and using it to discriminate unfairly. Third, we explore the increasing genetic surveillance of populations, and the potential costs for individual liberty.

Choosing better babies?

In the previous chapter, we explored the context in which women and men are making decisions to discover genetic information about themselves or their pregnancies, and we demonstrated how the rhetoric of choice concealed a lack of adequate information, and sometimes an insidious social pressure to avoid the birth of disabled children. But as well as this immediate context, there are wider social and cultural process driving individuals into screening out disability. Sometimes, this is to do with economic or legal pressures. For example, in countries where people depend on health insurance for assistance with care and medical costs for a disabled child, they might find it unavailable if they refuse to have prenatal tests or to terminate affected pregnancies. Philip Bereano notes that a pregnant woman in the USA whose foetus tested positive for cystic fibrosis was told by her health maintenance organization that it would pay for an abortion but would not cover the infant under the family's medical policy if she elected to carry the pregnancy to term.[1] Alternatively, health providers may insist on a whole battery of tests because they fear that otherwise they might face 'wrongful birth' suits from parents who have a disabled child. Although steps have been taken to prevent this, with various pieces of state and federal legislation, there are numerous examples of insurance companies flouting the law. At the same time, the poverty in which many disabled people find themselves, and the lack of opportunities for those who are not economically productive, make it much more difficult for parents to see the choice of having a disabled child as a positive one. Many disabled people and parents of disabled people report that the major difficulties with having an impairment are to do with restricted social choices and life chances. Increasingly, policy-makers may decide that the appropriate response to the disability problem is to screen prenatally, rather than to provide services and remove barriers to inclusion.

As well as these economic issues, there is often a cultural assumption that disability is a problem better avoided. For example, Marteau and Drake found that where women gave birth to people with Down's syndrome, having declined the opportunity to have prenatal screening, they were consequently more likely to be blamed for their situation.[2] Because many people are ignorant and fearful about disability, and because they find it impossible to imagine life as a disabled person, it is often suggested that it would be better to be dead than disabled. For this reason, people come to support prenatal screening, and also voluntary euthanasia.

Philosophers who might be expected to challenge superstition and prejudice often buy into the idea that disability is the worst thing that could happen to a person. For example, Glannon argues that we are morally required to terminate the development of embryos with genetic conditions that cause severe disease or disability because it is wrong to cause people to exist when pain and suffering would make their lives not worth living.[3] John Harris argues that deliberately producing children with more than slight disability is blameworthy.[4] US authors such as Buchanan and Brock have added to this literature on wrongful births and the harms to children whose parents declined screening.[5] Like some leading medical professionals and scientists in this field, these writers are adding to the pressure on women and men to terminate affected pregnancies.

Yet, in most cases, disability is not this sort of tragedy. There are instances of terrible suffering and early death from genetic disorders, and this is an area where some of these arguments may be justified. But the vast majority of disabled people do not experience such low quality of life. Where there is suffering associated with impairment, it is often more to do with restriction of social opportunities, not the consequences of a body or mind working in different ways: if society has caused the problem, then the imperative should be social change, not preventing the birth of the victim of social disadvantage. Otherwise we would be back to the eugenics of the past, where poor people were discouraged from reproducing, or we should advise minority ethnic communities that the problems of racism mean that they would be irresponsible to have children.

We recognize that in addition to social restrictions, many disabled people do experience physical problems consequent on their medical conditions. But these should be put into context. Every life involves a measure of suffering. This is not just one of the Buddha's Four Noble Truths, but also a statement of fact that may be uncomfortable but should be taken seriously. There are many things that are worse than impairment. Many non-disabled people have much more difficult lives than many disabled people. The problem is that the suffering associated with disability is seen as being more salient than other forms of difficulty. Yet many disabled people cope with their problems, life goes on, and their restrictions become irrelevant to them.

It should also be said that lots of disabled people don't suffer at all: their conditions do not involve pain or illness. People with sensory impairments or learning difficulties may be different, and may experience limitations, but they do not necessarily suffer as a result of their disability. Here philosophers are quick to label these forms of life inferior, or tragically limited. After all, a deaf person may never be able to enjoy Bach, a wheelchair user may never experience the exhilaration of reaching the summit of a mountain, and a person with Down's syndrome is unlikely to read the great works of literature. Only a philosopher would see the normal differences between individual lives as inherently problematic. In an ideal world, we would all exercise total choice and achieve whatever we wanted. Yet, in reality, most of us do lead limited lives, and do not experience everything that the world has to offer. It is true that blind people and people with intellectual limitations will miss out on some experiences. But these do not make their life not worth living, and there may even be compensatory advantages or possibilities.

Our views of what it is to be human, and how society should operate, need to be expanded by the reality of disability in our lives. If we take an individualistic view, and see life as a competitive struggle to succeed and prosper at all costs, then it is true that the disabled life may be inevitably inferior to the non-disabled life, and may be a cost to the rest of society. But if we follow a religious or humanistic perspective, then the value of life will rest in the relationships we have with one another. In his book *Becoming Human*, Jean Vanier argues that people with learning difficulties enable us all to be better human beings. We have to open up to the possibilities of living with difficulty, and valuing each other not for what we can make or sell, but because of our intrinsic worth and our social relationships. This perspective drove Vanier to found the L'Arche communities, where disabled people and non-disabled people live alongside each other, just as the philosophy of Rudolf Steiner led to the similar Camphill communities on a larger scale. Many people are disillusioned by the selfishness and shallow consumerism of the modern western world. These different ways of valuing individuals and each other not only challenge the eugenics associated with modern genetics, but also offer us ways forward out of our predicament.

The combination of individual choice, geneticization and new technology is driving us towards a future in which differences are not tolerated, and in which the responsibility for health is placed on the individual family, not on the wider social and economic institutions that generate ill-health. Elizabeth Beck-Gernsheim asks: 'Will the responsible parents of the future still be prepared to accept the fact that their child might have a handicap? Must they not rather do all in their power to make sure that no impairment exists?'[6] She outlines the ways in which these new technologies operate. Once a few people take advantage of new techniques, others feel disadvantaged if they do not have access to them, or if they do not take advantage of them. Slowly, a new standard is established. The new technique contributes to a further need, which was not there before. Parents are pressured to take up the test or treatment in a socially mobile society. A historic example of this is the rise in orthodontics and cosmetic surgery over the last two decades: it is no longer possible, in many areas of life, to be successful unless one has invested in good dentistry. The snaggle-teeth that were characteristic of previous generations are social disadvantages in the current one. Similarly, there is increasing pressure to conform by having cosmetic surgery, either to compensate for plainness or to remove the signs of ageing. The same process is at the heart of Lee Silver's account of *Remaking Eden*. He suggests that the combination of diagnostic power with in vitro fertilization will enable the increasing selection of embryos, not to avoid illness and impairment, but to choose better babies who will be more intelligent, beautiful and athletic. Elizabeth Beck-Gernsheim concludes: 'The technologies involved seem to be neutral. They threaten no one with extermination and destruction. They are not designed to help a "master race" to world domination. They do not disturb our good conscience. And so their attractiveness grows apace.'[7] The same arguments about promoting individual choice, and avoiding unnecessary suffering, will be used to justify these developments in the future. Given that they are likely to be costly interventions, they will not be available to all, and therefore they will increase social inequality.

Despite the hyperbole surrounding genetics, even with comprehensive screening some parents will give birth to disabled children. Most carrier tests will not detect all mutations and not all parents will undergo prenatal diagnosis. Moreover, there will always be disabled people because most impairment is not congenital, but is an outcome of ageing and accidents. Medical science is currently enabling people to live longer and longer. While quality of life will improve in older age, there will also be many more frail older people, many of whom may have impairments. Society must therefore accept disability and disabled people, not build a policy around elimination. Civil rights and social inclusion are vital, at every stage of the life cycle. Parents who decide to continue pregnancies affected by disability must be supported to do so as much as those who decide to have abortion. There is a danger that if genetic disease comes to be seen as always avoidable, as the current rhetoric of the Human Genome Project promises, parents of disabled children, carriers of genetic conditions and disabled people themselves may be socially isolated or stigmatized. As Hubbard comments,

> So once more, yes, a woman must have the right to terminate a pregnancy whatever her reasons, but she must also feel empowered not to terminate it, confident that the society will do what it can to enable her and her child to live fulfilling lives. To the extent that prenatal interventions implement social prejudices against people with disabilities they do not expand our reproductive choices. They constrict them.[8]

Welcome to the genetic underclass?

The decision to seek genetic information does not only affect individuals and their potential children. Because individuals share genetic characteristics with other family members, when people find things out about their susceptibilities to disease, this raises the question of their responsibility towards other family members. Should they warn their siblings about what they have discovered? The principle of privacy suggests that a person does not have an obligation to share genetic information with others. However, it could equally be argued that a person does have a responsibility to warn other people whom they know have a chance of being affected. For example, in the light of this information a person might want to change their behaviour to minimize their risk of contracting a particular disease. They might even want to reconsider the choice to have children. Many people affected by genetic disease do explain the implications to their relatives. Yet what about family members with whom they have lost contact or from whom they have been estranged? And what about relatives who might not wish to know their genetic susceptibilities, and prefer to remain ignorant? Conveying or not conveying genetic information may challenge or change family relationships.

While the ways in which genetics highlights changing notions of family and kinship are of interest and importance, many commentators have greater anxieties about access to genetic information by third parties outside the family. Genetic information is arguably different from other medical information because it is uniquely personal and it can be highly predictive. It therefore has considerable implications for employers and insurance companies. Such third parties may have vested interests in discovering the genetic make-up of individuals, and it is therefore particularly important to maintain confidentiality and genetic privacy, in order to avoid discrimination against people who have a genetic disposition to a particular disease and who might therefore be denied employment and insurance. For these reasons, the 1997 UNESCO Declaration on the Human Genome and Human Rights prohibits discrimination based on genetic characteristics (article 6) and promotes confidentiality of genetic data (article 7), while the Council of Europe's Convention on Biomedicine prohibits genetic discrimination (article 11) and upholds privacy – both the right to know, and the right not to know (article 10). Several American states have also introduced legislation restricting health insurance companies' access to genetic information. At the time of writing, President Bush has announced plans to protect genetic privacy, and the British government is also considering introducing legislation on this issue.

Many potential problems remain in this area. For example, there is no general concept of privacy in English law. Insurers can already demand access to medical records, and they have argued that genetic data are no different from existing medical tests and results, or information about family history. Insurance companies claim to be concerned that those at high risk of genetic diseases are disproportionately likely to take out health or life insurance. Conversely, those who find out that they are at low risk of disease may be less likely to take out insurance. This problem of 'adverse selection' may undermine the workings of the insurance market and drive up premiums. Certainly, the Association of British Insurers has stated that this is a concern. However, Professor Peter Harper argues that genetics need not create a problem for British insurers, and that the industry is wrong to insist on access to genetic test results.[9]

Insurance is meant to be a risk-spreading mechanism, and this depends on ignorance of the future. Insurance companies would like to be able to weight premiums as a result of genetic risk, just as they currently weight premiums depending on factors such as whether you smoke and where you live. This enables them to allocate applicants to different risk pools, members of which are charged the same premium: this is a mutuality model, and it depends on disclosure of relevant information. Hence insurers argue that disclosure of genetic information is the fairest way of running an insurance market. R. J. Pokorski, an industry representative, argues that it is not unfair to access genetic information: after all, this is already done crudely when applicants are required to fill out family profiles and undergo medical tests. Genetic data may actually benefit those who can be shown not to have an increased risk, despite other family or behavioural indications. Pokorski makes an argument for rational insurance criteria:

> Risk selection is properly performed and there is 'fair' discrimination when the applicant's expected future mortality and morbidity have been properly estimated and reflected in the premium rate. 'Unfair' discrimination, in contrast, is not and should not be permitted. Unfairness in the insurance context occurs when there is no sound actuarial justification for the manner in which risks are classified.[10]

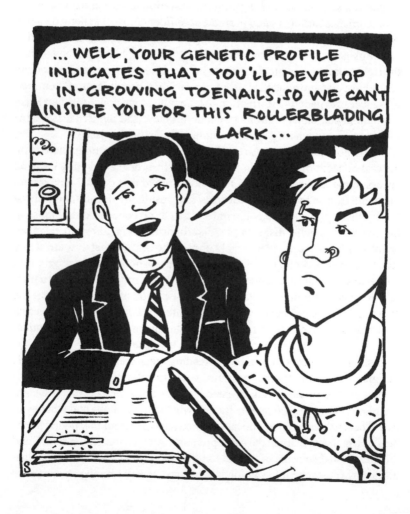

However, others have argued that both these types of discrimination should be prohibited. Hubbard and Wald argue that 'widespread use of genetic testing is bound to exacerbate the injustices inherent in for-profit health insurance'.[11] At present, in the UK, there is a voluntary prohibition on insurers asking for the results of genetic tests. Yet in practice, it would not be difficult for companies to get round regulation: for example, they could offer lower premiums to people who volunteer genetic information. Peter Harper argues that there is no need for insurers to require, or doctors to disclose, genetic test results for most normal life insurance and mortgage purposes: he proposes a ceiling, with only large life insurance applications needing genetic tests.[12] In any case, he argues that only dominant, late-onset conditions such as Huntington's disease could lead to adverse selection, because early-onset conditions would be obvious without the need for genetic testing. Even then, most single-gene disorders are extremely rare. For example, only about 200 cases of Huntington's disease are detected every year. Insuring people with these diseases could not seriously undermine the insurance industry.

The problem of genetics and insurance is particularly acute in the USA, where most people have private medical insurance. With the UK's collective social insurance system, everyone is covered by the NHS, everyone pays premiums via national insurance and taxation, and risk is pooled: the fact that some individuals are at higher genetic risk than others does not become a problem. This is called a solidarity model: everybody is included, and risk and benefit are distributed equally. In contrast, some commentators have suggested that the problem of genetic risk and negative selection will destroy the American insurance industry and force the development of a similar national health model. In the meantime many people with genetic diseases are suffering from discrimination, resulting in inadequate health care and even early mortality, as shown by a recent study comparing the life expectancy of people in the USA with cystic fibrosis who have private medical insurance cover and those who do not.[13]

There are also reasons to be wary of the extension of private health care in the UK. At present, some people, including members of the Labour government, have argued in favour of a greater role for the private insurance-based models for provision of health and welfare care in the UK. A report by the Institute for Public Policy Research suggested that this may raise problems in the context of greater powers of genetic prediction.[14] For example, insurance-based long-term care models for old age could be undermined or made inequitable when more genetic factors are discovered for degenerative conditions such as Alzheimer's and Parkinson's diseases: people with such predispositions could be priced out of the long-term care market, even though they may be at greatest need of such services.

Within the field of employment, there are similar dangers of genetic discrimination. Employers already have the right to select the most productive applicants, within legal constraints. Because genetics may be predictive of subsequent illness, actual or perceived genetic disease may lead to discrimination. A class of healthy people may be created, who are denied employment or restricted to lowly paid jobs because they may develop genetic diseases in midlife. This is already a problem in the USA, where health insurance comes as part of employment, and there is thus more incentive to screen workers.

But advocates of testing suggest reasons why testing of employees may be desirable. For example, particular occupations may expose individuals to hazards such as toxic chemicals. It may be in the interests of the employee to discover if they have a particular sensitivity to carcinogens or other hazards. The genetic condition alpha-antitrypsin deficiency predisposes people to the lung disease emphysema, especially if they are exposed to smoke or dust. In professions of high stress or responsibility – for example, in the armed forces or the airlines – ability to withstand altitude or fatigue or stress may be particularly important, and it may be desirable to exclude people who cannot operate at optimum efficiency. After all, they may put the public or their co-workers at risk.

However, it should be up to the individual to decide whether they wish to take particular tests, and not in the power of employers to force them to do so. Mass screening threatens people's autonomy and privacy. Proper counselling and support is unlikely to be provided. There are often difficulties in interpreting the results of occupational health screening. The particular role of genetic vulnerability may be minuscule compared to the gross dangers of pollution or other dangers affecting all workers. Genes always interact with the environment, so a higher priority should be to make the environment less polluting for everyone. While identification of some symptomatic workers is important, widespread workplace genetic screening is a dangerous rather than a beneficial development.

These are not simple scare stories. Evidence of dubious practices is already coming to light. For example, the Council for Responsible Genetics notes that in the USA Burlington Northern Santa Fe Railroad recently genetically tested employees for genes associated with carpal tunnel syndrome without their knowledge or consent, and threatened to sack at least one employee who refused to provide the blood sample until the US Equal Employment Opportunity Commission (EEOC) took it to court for violating the Americans with Disabilities Act. Without the activities of the Council for Responsible Genetics this might never have been exposed. It is too easy for employers and insurance companies to flout legislation. As Lenaghan notes, genetic diagnostics are developing fast, yet there are no proper legal safeguards to prevent discrimination in the UK, and the American legislation is complex and difficult to enforce.[15]

Bartha Knoppers has proposed several safeguards in order to avoid genetic discrimination in employment.[16] Existing anti-discrimination legislation such as the Disability Discrimination Act in the USA could include the prevention of discrimination against people who are perceived as being disabled due to being carriers or having presymptomatic conditions. Yet she accepts that job-related pre-employment genetic testing should be allowed with individuals' consent. Instead of advocating a ban on this practice she calls for a national agency to control testing. This would rely on a principle of corporate solidarity to govern use of genetic information, and socially responsible behaviour by industry. This emphasis on partnership between state and industry, self-regulation and industry access to 'relevant' genetic information is characteristic of many of the policy discussions in this arena. Such arguments display a startling naivety, given that industry so often puts profit before morality, produces weak and flexible self-imposed regulation, and systematically flouts state regulation that is difficult to enforce.

Despite our qualms about the proliferation of genetic testing, which we discussed in the previous chapter, we should also note that there is a danger that the fear of discrimination might discourage people from having genetic tests. Professor John Burn has suggested that 'If insurance companies are allowed access to genetic information people may avoid taking genetic tests that could save their lives for fear of not getting a mortgage or life insurance. Insurance companies will in effect be killing people.'[17] Although the potential for genetic cures is far from obvious, and the dangers of systematic surveillance or surgical intervention should be acknowledged, there are obviously cases where a genetic diagnosis can be a benefit to people's health. Troy Duster and Diane Beeson's research with families with cystic fibrosis in the USA has found evidence of people concealing their cystic fibrosis status from their health care practitioner where their symptoms are relatively mild and can be treated in their own terms, for example as a chronic chest infection, because of fears of stigma and discrimination by employers or insurance companies. They note:

> Adults with CF who can avoid being officially diagnosed or labeled often do so to avoid discrimination. We interviewed a relative of two adults with CF who are hiding their diagnosis. One is in the military, and the other is a professional who seeks treatment out of state because he fears his career will be jeopardized if his condition is known. Neither of these adults would agree to be interviewed due to fears of disclosure of

their conditions. In both cases employability, and more indirectly, health care coverage are concerns.[18]

This kind of non-disclosure may well mean that people are denied comprehensive treatments and care which could be of real health benefit. More generally, survey research reveals that consumers may well be reluctant to take genetic tests for these reasons: one poll found that 30 per cent of people would not take a genetic test if faced with a disclosure requirement.[19] As well as the danger of people being discouraged from taking tests, there is also the problem of people being forced to take tests, even if they wish to remain ignorant of their genetic status, in order to get insurance or employment. And as always, there is a danger that such testing procedures may be inaccurate, or may take place in the absence of appropriate communication and counselling support.

Of course, it should be noted that the results of many genetic tests are very vague, and would thus be of little help to insurance companies, or relevance to employers. While presymptomatic tests for conditions like Huntington's disease could be of great interest to employers and insurers, tests showing slight predispositions to complex polygenic disorders will be less relevant, but might lead to unfair discrimination. Equally, we might see a repeat of the 1970s sickle cell controversy, with carriers also facing discrimination from employers and insurers. Finally, where testing is demanded during pregnancy, insurance considerations may cause pressure for termination of pregnancy, removing the right of women to choose whether to continue a pregnancy affected by genetic abnormality.

Our survey of the issues suggests that the new genetic information will be a mixed blessing for most people. In the many cases where considerable uncertainty surrounds genetic results, knowledge will increase, not decrease, stress. Where people discover they are likely to develop a disease for which there is no treatment or a poor prognosis, stress will inevitably result. Where information concerns susceptibility, individuals may fail to follow health advice, or may feel fatalistic about their chances. In all cases, privacy, consent and control of information are vitally important, but particularly in the contexts of insurance and employment.

Other medical tests have also been surrounded by controversy, such as HIV tests. But genetic tests are different from most other medical investigations because of their predictive power, and because of their implications for other family members. Yet samples for genetic testing can be easily obtained. Saliva traces, sweat or hair could be gathered by a third party without the knowledge or consent of the person being tested. This shows the significance of the new era of genetic information that we are entering. In the field of health care itself, we concur with the views of geneticists and commentators such as Peter Harper, Angus Clarke and Abby Lippman that many proposed screening programmes will be highly costly, will bring few benefits and will generate new risks and problems for individuals and society.

Towards the surveillance society

In the final part of this chapter, we widen our focus to look at the new social tendencies towards the use of genetic information for surveillance of citizens, and the discourses of risk and responsibility that arise from new forms of genetic knowledge and new claims about genetic factors in social behaviours. Here we are linking three separate areas. First, we discuss the ways in which individuals are made increasingly responsible for their own health, and often that of their families, via knowledge of genetic risks. Second, we discuss the use of DNA fingerprinting and police access to genetic information. Third, we explore the debate about 'biological culpability' and the use of behavioural genetics markers to predict individuals at risk of committing crime. These disparate areas of social policy are connected by the theme of surveillance, prevention and responsibility. They also point to an irony: at the outset of medical sociology, the American functionalist Talcot Parsons distinguished illness as that form of deviance from social rules for which an individual could not be held responsible, as opposed to crime, a form of deviance to which blame could be attached. Fifty years later, we may see illness as something that an individual needs to take responsibility for avoiding, whereas it is argued that some forms of crime may be determined by genetic or neurological factors beyond an individual's control.

Genetic risks

We have already begun to highlight the ways in which genetics makes individuals responsible for their own health and that of their families. Prospective parents are encouraged to have a battery of screening tests to ensure that their baby will not have a genetic condition. When individuals are found to be at risk of a genetic disease, they bear two sorts of responsibility. The first is to avoid behaviours likely to exacerbate that risk. This starts with consulting and following the advice of medical experts. People may have to submit to regular screening tests and check-ups, to change their diet, to avoid particular risky behaviours. This development could be seen as part of a broader approach to health promotion, where individual factors are prioritized over wider social and economic factors such as poverty, working conditions, bad housing and other forms of deprivation. Rather than health behaviours being placed in a broader cultural and social context, individuals are blamed for their bad diet, or their use of alcohol or nicotine.[20]

Second, individuals bear responsibility for informing their genetic kin about their risk. Nina Hallowell's research with women with genetic risk of breast and ovarian cancer shows how seriously these responsibilities are taken.[21] They talked about putting other people's needs before their own, about their obligation to encourage family members to undergo screening, about their duty to take part in research and clinical trials. In particular, they talked about their responsibility towards their children to take all steps possible to avoid falling ill, and failing in their maternal responsibilities.

The drive to identify genetic elements in illness has moved beyond rare diseases such as the inherited forms of breast and ovarian cancer into the everyday diseases such as dementia, diabetes and hypertension which many people suffer in later life. In order to develop knowledge of these complex multi-factorial conditions, vast amounts of data are needed from a broad section of the population. While the route to finding the breast cancer or Huntington's genes was to find families where many members had suffered these diseases, the route to identifying genes of small effect in these complex diseases is to take samples and medical information from hundreds of thousands of individuals. The databanks arising from such research may be able to help with the development of pharmaco-genetics, in which more precisely targeted pharmaceuticals are deployed to halt or delay the onset of the major degenerative diseases.

While there are many population genetic databanks in existence, collections on the vast scale needed for this new research are only now being developed and planned. For example, a highly controversial project has led to the genetic and medical data of the entire population of Iceland being gathered by a commercial company, deCode Genetics. Iceland is of particular interest because it has a small population that is thought to be ethnically homogenous (although this is now doubtful), and because comprehensive medical records have been kept there for many generations. Other small nations, such as Estonia, are currently auctioning access to their population databanks. In the UK, the Medical Research Council and the Wellcome Trust have proposed a major population genetic database covering approximately half a million individuals.

Various ethical and social questions are raised by these vast extensions in surveillance, some of which led the Icelandic Medical Council to declare: 'The [ethical] committee is completely opposed to the present bill and will advise Icelandic physicians not to participate in the setting up of the database.'[22] The first concern with such databanks is about confidentiality. In order to make the best use of genetic information, information about health experience and behaviour is also needed. Therefore, the genetic samples have to be connected, in some way, to the health records of the individuals. As the Medical Research Council in the UK suggested,

> Databases of genetic information can be anonymised, but for much medical research, including that on the genetic factors affecting disease risk or response to treatment, it must be possible to link individual data to names, contact addresses or other information that can identify individuals in order that the database can be updated with follow-up surveys about people's health and lifestyle from time to time.[23]

This means that there is a risk of third parties discovering important genetic information, which can lead to discrimination, as we have seen earlier. People may be deterred from having genetic tests or consulting their doctor because of fears of this occurring.

Some advocates of the genetic databank point to possible direct benefits for individuals taking part: researchers may be able to tell them about their genetic susceptibilities. Yet this reinforces the danger of private information becoming public property. It also potentially undermines the individual's right not to know what illnesses they may succumb to in later life. And there is a risk that information will not be communicated in the context of proper support and counselling.

The second major problem with genetic databanks is commercial exploitation. Biotechnology companies will be directly involved with population databases, as in Iceland, or will have close relationships with the projects, as in the UK. If pharmaceuticals are to be developed as a result of genetic databases, then it will be commercial organizations that do this work and take the profits. Although the Icelandic population have been promised free drugs developed as a result of their databank, profit rather than altruism drives companies in this sector. As more people's data are accessed, more nations and more pharmaceutical companies become involved in this sector of genomics, and more treatments are developed, free drugs for donors are an unlikely scenario.

Third, as we have argued above, genetic databanking is part of a tendency to focus on the individual genetic elements in health, rather than broader social and environmental factors. On a global scale, we should point out that 90 per cent of medical research is carried out on diseases that affect 10 per cent of the world's population, with 50 per cent of all health spending being carried out in the USA, which has just 5 per cent of the world's population. There is a strong argument that research and health care are needed on the easily preventable diseases that currently cause premature death and suffering in the majority world, not on the late-onset and lifestyle-related diseases of the affluent minority.

Policing by genetics

Outside the medical sphere, DNA databases are already in use in many western countries. Since its first application in 1983, the use of genetic fingerprinting has become a major tool for modern police forces, and has enabled detectives to solve major crimes including rape and murder, as well as everyday offences such as burglary. The majority of the population are supportive of the use of DNA fingerprinting. After all, if you haven't done anything wrong, there's nothing to worry about. And who could argue with efficient detection of criminals, as well as the possible deterrence effects of this new forensic technique?

Yet a number of problems are raised by this new form of genetic surveillance. First, there are questions about the accuracy of the process. Efficiency dictates that the entire genome is not the unit of identification. Instead, a small number of separate polymorphisms, called SNIPs – differences in DNA – are examined. If the suspect's DNA coincides with the crime scene sample on these different SNIPs, then there is a very high probability that they were the original source of the sample. Yet different sub-populations differ slightly in their DNA make-up. While a particular SNIP may be very rare in the population at large, it might be relatively common in an ethnic minority group. Therefore the likelihoods are always relative to the population surveyed. But this can easily be overlooked in the search for certainty.

Equally, there are possibilities for error in the process of taking samples and recording results. Inefficiency or incompetence could result in the guilty avoiding detection, or the innocent being framed. A study in 1993 of 45 American laboratories found that in 18 out of 223 tests, a match was identified where it did not exist.[24] Because it is easy to obtain personal samples – for example, hair or skin cells – it is theoretically possible for an innocent individual's genetic material to be left at a crime scene. Whether by accident or design, DNA fingerprinting is not infallible. But many people do not understand the risk of laboratory error. In a court of law, DNA evidence may have irrefutable scientific status: it may sway a jury to convict because it appears to be modern, objective and powerful.

Second, there are civil liberties questions over the collection and retention of DNA samples. While few people would object to samples being taken from those found guilty of a serious offence, many may think it wrong to retain a sample from someone who was found not guilty, or who was involved in non-violent crimes. But these limitations are often breached. In the USA in 1990, Congress funded a programme to take biological samples from all military personnel, mainly to identify dead bodies in conflict situations. Service personnel refusing to be tested were court-martialled. These military DNA data are also available to law enforcement services. Some American states allow their police DNA databanks to be used in paternity proceedings. DNA evidence is widely used by the FBI: for example, they analysed saliva on postage stamps to identify a suspect in the 1993 World Trade Center attack and the Unabomber.

In 1989, the British government allowed immigration officials to use DNA identification tests for immigration applicants who claimed to have relatives in the UK: 18,000 tests have since been carried out, often in a racially discriminatory manner. Since 1995, the British police have collected nearly a million profiles from those suspected, cautioned, charged or convicted of crimes: about 6,000 new samples are added every week. And although profiles are meant to be removed if you are later acquitted of a crime, there's evidence that this isn't happening. Coneas gives an estimate of about 50,000 illegal retentions of information in the UK Forensic DNA database.[25] If you are found guilty, your data are on record until you die. Some commentators fear that the police are building up a comprehensive database by stealth: by 2004, it will contain records of 3 million people. This may well be a benefit in solving some crimes, but it is also an invasion of privacy and a major increase in state surveillance.

Third, there are potential links between medical and forensic uses of genetic information. For example, there was a case in Glasgow of an individual taking part in a medical trial whose data were passed to police for forensic purposes. And there are fears that the SNIPs used for DNA fingerprinting may also convey information about genetic predispositions of the individual, which should remain confidential. For example, one SNIP is close to a marker used to indicate diabetes susceptibility.[26] As diagnostic techniques become more powerful in the future, vast quantities of information could potentially be revealed by police DNA samples, via the use of gene chip technology. The Wellcome/MRC database proposal suggests that individual patient records, which the NHS is planning to computerize in the near future, will be linked to the research database. There may be a risk of blurring the line between these records and police forensic investigations. After all, at present the police already have the right to consult an individual's medical case-notes.

The genetics of criminal behaviour

The third and final area of genetic surveillance moves further into the domain of criminality. This is the potential for testing or screening for a genetic predisposition to criminal behaviour. We have already cast doubt on the validity of genetic explanations of this type. But we should also recognize their seductive powers, and the possibilities for techniques being developed in this area despite the dubiety of the evidence on which they are based. There is a long and dubious tradition of biologically based explanations of criminality, notoriously in the case of Lombroso: this work has often had racist overtones. Social scientists have rejected the idea that there are biological factors in crime. Yet according to its advocates, the modern behavioural genetics has provided scientific data rather than prejudice and pseudo-scientific theories.

There are two parts to the contemporary argument about the biology of crime. The first suggests that particular individuals are less able to control their behaviour due to genetic, neurological or hormonal differences from the rest of the population. This raises the question of whether offenders with such differences can be held responsible for their actions in the same way as the rest of the population. There have been a number of attempts in American and British court cases to deny culpability, or to reduce charges from murder to manslaughter, or to use a defence of temporary insanity. These legal defences have drawn on research about families with a seemingly inherited predisposition to violence, or pre-menstrual syndrome, or other biological processes. However, there have been few successful claims of biology as an excuse or justification for criminality: the judicial process has been very resistant to enabling individuals to evade responsibility for their actions.[27]

The second area of debate concerns the value of behavioural genetic or neuroscientific research in predicting individuals at risk of violent or criminal behaviour, and potentially enabling them to have educational or psychological or even pharmaceutical interventions to prevent them offending. Research reveals a concordance between the offending behaviour of identical twins which suggests that shared genes may have an effect. Behavioural geneticists are not suggesting that there is a single gene for criminality, and are not denying the importance of upbringing and environment. Nor do they generally make claims about differences between ethnic groups, confining their research to differences between individuals. However, they claim that there may be a number of genes of small effect that interact to increase the risk of anti-social behaviour, for example.

These claims are extremely contentious. The negative social effects on individuals of being diagnosed as potential criminals might outweigh any possible positive effects of education or therapy. The idea of prescribing pharmaceuticals to healthy, innocent individuals raises major civil liberties questions: the existing trend in American classrooms towards prescribing the psychoactive drug Ritalin to large numbers of children who supposedly have attention deficit hyperactivity disorder (ADHD) is already of major concern.[28] In the case of potentially violent or anti-social individuals – as currently in the case of those identified as being paedophiles or schizophrenics – there may well be calls for preventative detention, electronic tagging or other surveillance. All these suggestions for utilizing the new data emerging from behavioural genetics challenge our social notions of free will and determinism, as well as the place of freedom in liberal societies, and they potentially lead to the creation of a whole range of 'risky identities'. As Nikolas Rose concludes, 'Biological criminology, here, is but one element in the more general rise of public health strategies of crime control, focusing on the identification of, and preventative intervention upon, aggressive, risky or monstrous anti-citizens.'[29]

Conclusion

This review of the consequences of genetic testing and screening has focused upon the pressure to eliminate disabled foetuses, the potential for the intensification of discrimination and stigma against disabled people and the growing trend of genetic surveillance of people's health and behaviour. In the previous chapter, we outlined the way in which information and choice about genetic testing and screening are restricted by a range of cultural values and social pressures as well as by uncertainties within genetic knowledge itself. These aspects of contemporary genomics are different from the eugenics of the past, in that coercion is less explicit and discrimination is more covert. A range of commercial companies, employers and insurance companies, in particular, are discriminating on the basis of genetic information, and the state is involved in pushing forward genetic screening and surveillance in the interests of public health and public safety. All of these practices have echoes of the past which simplistic appeals to choice and equity do not dampen, given the gap between professional rhetoric and the reality of people's experiences.

We have also highlighted several features of what has been aptly called the 'slippery slope' towards a deeper and more profound form of eugenics: more genetic tests and screening programmes for more and more conditions gathered under the genetic label, and more expectation that people will comply with these tests as commercial companies sell their services and additional genetic tests are 'bolted on' to existing services in national health care systems. This suggests that robust and far-reaching regulation is necessary to prevent the intensification of eugenic practices. But contemporary regulation of genomics is far from adequate. In the next chapter we explore why this is the case.

10

Regulating genomics

The new genetics is regulated through a complex series of laws, treaties and codes of practice, which affect the activities of the professionals and organizations that are involved in research and clinical provision. Much of the legislation is not specific to genetics, affecting medicine, science and the use of information in a general sense. In the UK, examples of this legislation might include the Medicines Control Act or the regulations governing the use of animals in scientific research. Recently the growth of human genomics, and associated research involving embryo stem cells and cloning, has prompted increased interest in the global regulation of genetic medicine and science. Organizations that are part of the United Nations, such as UNESCO and the World Health Organization, have drafted treaties and guidelines on genetics, as has the European Union. Scientists' own organizations, such as HUGO and the Society of Clinical Geneticists, also have guidelines on the use of genetic information by third parties, patient confidentiality, informed choice in genetic counselling, and so on. But national governments have been reluctant to introduce specific legislation to curtail ethically problematic practices related to genetics. Even when legislation is in place, it is fairly limited. For example, American law restricts the use of genetic information by government employers, not the commercial sector. And the British Human Fertilisation and Embryology Act restricts research to organizations approved by a licensing authority (dominated by professionals). Instead, governments rely heavily on self-regulation on the part of industry and the professional scientists, clinicians and allied professionals involved in the field. A variety of non-statutory commissions and committees perform this role, through various public consultations and the issuing of reports and recommendations, but geneticists and allied professionals dominate their membership.

Supranational treaties and self-regulation are the mainstay of contemporary regulation of genetics. Without them we might well be faced with a kind of regulatory vacuum around genetics, given national governments' deference to commerce and science. But these forms of regulation are often ineffective and anti-democratic, putting the interests of the professions before the interests of patients and society at large. The recent emphasis on regulatory transparency and accountability, through open consultation with the public, should also be treated with scepticism, given that criticisms are sidelined and consultations are carefully managed to support the professional consensus.

There are several reasons for this climate of soft regulation. The neoliberal emphasis on medico-scientific progress and individual rights means that restrictions on research are considered to be backward and restrictions on access to genetic tests or screening would be viewed as discriminatory. Regulation therefore tends to support the expansion of genetic research and services. Coupled to this emphasis on rights is a burgeoning rhetoric of personal responsibility for health and welfare. In order to engage in individual governance, people must be able and willing to access genetic tests and modify their lifestyles accordingly, and genetic services must expand to service this desire. Professionals are also expected to act responsibly, through self-regulation, peer-review and involvement in non-statutory regulatory committees and commissions. It is not surprising that their inclination is towards expansion of genetic research and services and further devolution of regulation, rather than the imposition of what they would view as restrictive legislation. Bioethicists, whose regulatory role is also flourishing, tend to be equally enamoured of individual rights and medical progress, and their contribution fits well with the paradigm of abuse prevention so favoured by professionals and governments.

Allied to the rise of neoliberalism, the market is increasingly important in shaping the regulation of the genome. Consumer rights are valued above citizen rights, which effectively means that the rights of well-resourced and able-bodied health consumers to genetic tests take precedence over the rights of disabled people to equality. The commercial environment in which genetic and associated research is increasingly conducted also makes it very difficult for governments to regulate their practices. One favoured route, restricting state funds to set the research agenda, does not touch the commercial sector. And the important role of biotechnology and pharmaceutical companies in the national and international economies makes even the most powerful contemporary states back off from more restrictive patent legislation. International co-operation on robust regulation is also unlikely, when national economic interests weigh heavily on policy-making representatives. The increasingly global nature of commercial biotechnology and genomics also means that even the most ethically dubious practices, like human cloning, cannot be globally banned. Even when global treaties are in place, their wording is often deliberately vague and flexible to cater for different national interests, and restrictions are therefore weak and often ineffectual.

In this chapter we focus upon the activities of the state at a national and international level, considering treaties and protocols as well as laws and guidelines concerning genetic research, genetic services and genetic discrimination. We are particularly concerned by the relationship between the state and the market, the devolution of decision making to professionals, and the rise of institutional bioethics as a regulatory tool. We also discuss more recent efforts to take account of public opinion in policy making, in order to assess whether this might point the way to more democratic and robust regulatory practices.

Regulatory bioethics

As Jonsen has noted in *The Birth of Bioethics*, bioethics grew out of post-war concerns about medical ethics in the new medicine and biology, including concerns about the quality of the gene pool, expressed by geneticists such as Herman J. Muller, as discussed previously.[1] Philosophers, theologians, lawyers and social scientists joined the various centres of study that were set up in the USA in the 1960s, as bioethics began to institutionalize. Around the same time, the federal government became interested in bioethics associated with genetic engineering, transplantation, and research involving human subjects and foetal tissue, and set up various commissions to investigate these issues.

In these discussions and hearings three fundamental principles of bioethics emerged: respect for persons, beneficence and justice. When applied to human genetics, bioethicists and scientists discussed the ethical obligations of genetic counsellors to remain neutral, versus their commitment not to do harm; and weighed up the benefits to society of abortion of defective foetuses, versus the rights of the individual to informed choice, and the rights of people already living with disabilities. Genetic therapy was also discussed in terms of costs and benefits to society and the individual. Jonsen's description of one report published in 1981 captures this well: '*Screening and Counselling for Genetic Conditions* endorsed programs for genetic screening, counseling and education [based on the principles of] preservation of confidentiality, respect for personal autonomy, improved knowledge about genetics, provision of benefit and equity in access.'[2] Another important report, produced the following year, *Splicing Life*, was instrumental in drawing a distinction between germ line and somatic gene therapy. The British inquiry into embryo research and assisted reproduction (discussed in Chapter 6) was also important in setting the ethical standards on which this work should be based, rejecting commercialization and sanctioning research on foetuses less than 14 days old.

The American and British governments responded to these commissions and inquiries by producing several pieces of legislation. The USA tended towards restricting state funds to research that complied with the government's ethical prescriptions. The UK tended to favour the establishment of licensing or oversight authorities to certify and monitor scientific and medical practices. State interference was unattractive, especially in the realms of medicine or commerce. The professionals who were instrumental in the establishment of these restrictions therefore dominated licensing authorities and oversight bodies. This effectively constituted state-sanctioned self-regulation. The state and the profession took on the role of standard setting, facilitating the expansion of legitimate genetic services that were perceived to be in the public interest.

Bioethics as a discipline also developed a distinct line of thinking about genetics. Notwithstanding the high media profile of utilitarian bioethicists like Peter Singer and John Harris, for the most part bioethicists reject old-style eugenics and utilitarianism in favour of respect for the individual and medico-scientific progress in curing disease. But echoes of both eugenics and utilitarianism still suffuse bioethical discussions of genetics, within a framework that privileges the individual who wants to 'do good'. As we have already discussed, individual choice is often used as an argument for the expansion of genetic services. Embryo research and therapeutic cloning are justified in terms of the benefits they will bring to people with genetic diseases. In both cases it is assumed that the interests of the sick individual and society in the 'good life' are the same.

We would therefore argue that although bioethics has been important in excluding some of the most extreme forms of eugenics, it has also been party to the opening of what Troy Duster has described as the backdoor to eugenics. This is well illustrated in the following quote by Caplan and colleagues:

> No moral principle seems to provide sufficient reason to condemn individual eugenic goals. While force and coercion, compulsion and threat have no place in procreative choice, and while individual decisions can have negative collective consequences, it is not clear that it is any less ethical to allow parents to pick the eye colour of their child or to try and create a fetus with a propensity for mathematics than it is to permit them to teach their children the values of a particular religion, try to inculcate a love of sports by taking them to football games, or to require them to

play the piano. In so far as coercion and force are absent and individual choice is allowed to hold sway, then presuming fairness in the access to the means of enhancing our offspring's lives it is hard to see what exactly is wrong with parents choosing to use genetic knowledge to improve the health and well-being of their offspring.[3]

Here the principles of individual choice and equity of access are used as arguments for genetic enhancement and the selection of behavioural and physical characteristics; practices that are equated with learning and socialization of children. Caplan and colleagues ignore the subtle and not so subtle ways in which individuals' decisions in favour of enhancement and selection would be influenced by stigma and discrimination in society, and they give scant regard to the intensification of discrimination that these decisions would engender. The political economy of medical science is also ignored and the value of so-called scientific progress is unquestioned. This kind of abstract rationalization is not only naïve and misleading, it is dangerous, because it justifies eugenics by appealing to a burgeoning neoliberal doctrine of rights and choice.

Another reason to be wary of bioethics is its alignment with the genetics establishment. Bioethics can lend respectability to genetics without challenging its fundamental strategies, or promoting more rigorous forms of control and audit of research and clinical services. For example, the Ethical Legal and Social Implications (ELSI) programme allied to the Human Genome Project has been heavily criticised for failing to tackle fundamental problems such as the commercialization of the genome. This judgement is a little harsh, given that the ELSI scholars have, to a large extent, been constrained by the political and economic context of genomics. And we should remember that they have nevertheless produced some important work. For example, Annas's draft bill on genetic discrimination was influential in the formulation of legislation banning genetic discrimination in federal workplaces. But there is no doubt that the Human Genome Project has forged ahead, with bioethics safely cordoned off in the ELSI programme.

More generally, bioethics has provided scientists and doctors with an agreeable ethical code that does little to challenge their practices and professional values. Bioethics came to be valued in genetics because it applied abstract reasoning and precise definition to particular situations and questions that these new technologies and forms of knowledge posed, valuing informed choice, scientific progress and equity of access to genetic services. This provided scientists and doctors with a technical language and thought-style which suits their professional values, whilst at the same time providing a route into wider discussions about the impact of their work; discussions in which geneticists want to play a central part. Of course, it would be wrongheaded to criticize scientists and doctors for grappling with the ethics of their work, but we must be wary of the powerful alliance of professionals who have successfully promoted this narrow form of bioethics, to the exclusion of more sophisticated and challenging ethical discussion and policy. This can be seen at the international, national and professional levels, as we now go on to discuss.

Treaties and protocols at international and national levels

UNESCO's Universal Declaration on the Human Genome and Human Rights (adopted on 11 November 1997) was among the first international guidelines to be produced on the human genome. The declaration emphasizes the right of the individual to respect for their dignity and rejects genetic determinism. It seeks a balance between ethical concerns and scientific progress, supporting genetic services for serious diseases with proper counselling services, but rejecting reproductive cloning. The World Health Organization's *Proposed International Guidelines on Ethical Issues in Medical Genetics and Genetic Services* (1998) take a similar stance, favouring genetic services based around the principles of informed choice, confidentiality, equity of access and public education about genetics. Bioethicists and geneticists had a leading role in the formulation of these guidelines, which, although they are non-binding, take crucial steps towards an emergent global bioethics on genetics. Once more we can see that respect for the individual forms a central plank of the resolutions, which steer a careful course around difficult issues to promote an international consensus. This has led to accusations of blandness, but compromise was essential if these guidelines were to have any impact on practices and policy making in nation states.

The firmest statements of censure at an international level concern human cloning. For example, following the furore over Dolly the sheep, the World Health Assembly rejected cloning to replicate humans as 'ethically unacceptable and contrary to human dignity and morality'. But the ethicists and professionals who dominate the international commissions tend to shy away from what they see as knee-jerk responses to scientific developments, and prefer a more measured response on issues such as these, emphasizing the benefits of therapeutic cloning.[4]

The European regulatory framework is equally conservative. For example, the European Convention for Human Rights and Biomedicine

(April 1997) seeks to shield the individual from threats from society. Although it recognizes the benefits to humanity from genetic research and services, it states that the rights of human beings are of paramount importance. The convention prohibits discrimination on the grounds of genetic heritage, including predictive testing for reasons other than health or related research. It also states that intervention in the human genome must be for preventative, diagnostic or therapeutic reasons, not for enhancement of the genome. But the convention is vague about the use of genetic tests by insurance companies where the test has already been performed and the individual consents to passing on the information to their insurer. The prohibition on human cloning (added in 1998) is also vague, leaving it up to individual countries to decide what 'human being' means. And the convention is not mandatory, which means that countries like the UK, where this kind of research takes place, have simply declined to sign it.

Another European body that makes pronouncements on genetics is the European Group on Ethics in Science and New Technologies (EGESNT). It holds round table discussions and publishes 'opinions' in an effort to guide ethical debate on controversial topics. One example of a recent opinion published by the group concerns the Ethical Aspects of Human Stem Cell Research and Use (14 November 2000). The standard ethical principles of respect for human dignity, individual autonomy, justice, beneficence and freedom of research guided their conclusions. Proportionality, where research methods are necessary to the aims pursued and no alternative more acceptable methods are available, and precaution, where unintended consequences must be borne in mind, were also highlighted in the report. This means that its conclusions are very consistent with an emergent national and international consensus on the use of stem cells, where commercialization and the creation of embryos for research purposes are considered problematic, but the use of discarded embryos for research is justified according to risk–benefit evaluation. The group also favours centralized licensing authorities in member countries, modelled on the British Human Fertilization and Embryology Authority (HFEA).

Although we must welcome these careful ethical considerations, and the important role of bioethicists in challenging the dominance of professional geneticists in regulation at the international level, their approach and conclusions are often disappointing. Their role is declarative rather than legislative, and as such they are fairly weak. The application of a standard set of moral rules and techniques for balancing different interests, and the dominance of concern for the right of the individual in these decisions, also tend towards a particularly conservative and uniform set of precepts. Boundaries between so-called therapeutic and reproductive cloning, somatic and germ-line therapy, and disease and behaviour, are narrowly defined and impose an artificial divide between practices and knowledge, which are in fact increasingly blurred. Neither are the social context and implications of individual choices properly addressed. This, alongside concerns to respect moral pluralism among member countries, means that ethical rulings lack a progressive and critical edge, and give over too much to scientific progress, failing to staunch the commercialization, discrimination and human cloning they are so keen to avoid. The involvement of a wider range of constituencies in these decision-making bodies, including those who challenge the alliance of institutional bioethics and professional geneticists, would provoke more sophisticated and challenging policy making, as would consultation with a broader range of groups concerned by the new genetics. However, the fundamentally conservative nature of these bodies and groupings means that ethical activism about the genome must also be located elsewhere for it to have any radical impact on policy and practice.

National non-statutory advisory bodies

Non-statutory advisory bodies have also proliferated in the era of the genome, particularly in the UK. The British government (including the Conservative administration of John Major, 1992–7, and the Labour administration of Tony Blair, 1997 to the present) has established various commissions to look into genetics, although it tends to ignore their recommendations when they do not fit with its neoliberal ideology of public–private partnership, personal responsibility and consumer choice. The Human Genetics Advisory Commission's recommendation of a moratorium on insurance companies' use of genetic information was ignored by the Blair government in 1997, in favour of the industry's much maligned code of practice and the establishment of yet another licensing committee, the Genetics and Insurance Advisory Committee. Its more recent incarnation, the Human Genetics Commission (HGC) has tended to be quite cautious in its pronouncements about genetic testing and information (perhaps wary of its own demise should it be too critical, like its predecessor), although it has recently joined the House of Commons Science and Technology Committee's criticism of the insurance industry, and called for legislation to restrict insurance companies' access to genetic information. The government is apparently proceeding with this, although the legislative timetable is still unclear. The HGC has also been critical of the government's plans to extend the national DNA database, the police forensic database, to include DNA samples from everyone suspected of a crime – even those for whom the charges are subsequently dropped – and has raised concerns about the use of such a database for predictive testing.

These critical salvos are not as out of character as they might first appear. They are, in fact, understandable when we consider that they represent the mainstream views of geneticists who tend to see insurance companies' use of genetic information as a barrier to the extension of genetic tests, and who view behavioural genetics and state-sanctioned surveillance with suspicion. Lawyers on the HGC undoubtedly share geneticists' suspicions about state surveillance and interest in prediction of criminality, given their own experiences of the criminal justice system. But these criticisms must also be set in the wider international and national context of a more usually supportive approach to genetic science and medicine, emphasizing the usual triumvirate of individual choice, equitable access to genetic services and medico-scientific progress.

Support for genetics is also reflected in the membership of these various committees, which are overwhelming dominated by scientists, doctors and bioethicists (including philosophers, theologians and lawyers). Very few lay people are represented on commissions and committees of this type, and even those who are can often be considered 'professional lay people', in the sense that they have made a career out of committee membership. Some critics are present, like Dr Bill Albert who represents the International Committee of the British Council of Disabled People on the HGC, but they are few and far between, and must always be wary of the danger of tokenism. The Genetics and Insurance Committee (GAIC) is one of the worst examples of skewed committee membership, with some of its members nominated by the Association of British Insurers (ABI) and the Institute of Actuaries. The geneticist Sandy Raeburn advises the ABI and is its representative on the GAIC. Although this is a situation that many geneticists in the public sector deplore, and it is these geneticists who are by far the most influential in terms of policy making in the UK for the time being, the alliance between geneticists and commerce will inevitably grow as the pharmacogenomics and proteomics sectors develop. The GAIC has been heavily criticized by the House of Commons Science and Technology Select Committee, but we remain doubtful about a radical overhaul of its membership or remit, and wary about the growing influence of the market on policy making, as we shall discuss shortly.

Skewed membership, a narrow technical remit and the ideologies of scientific progress and individual choice are also reflected in the various satellite advisory bodies who influence policy more indirectly, such as the British Nuffield Council on Bioethics. Funded by the Nuffield Foundation, the Wellcome Trust and the Medical Research Council, the Nuffield Council considers the ethical issues arising from developments in medicine and biology. Its report, *Genetic Screening: Ethical Issues* (1993) emphasized informed consent, easy access to services, confidentiality and government oversight of genetic services and their implications – the standard diet of regulation. It also favoured genetic screening of employees and the use of genetic data by insurance companies in specific situations, to be established by other regulatory bodies, where the disease is well characterized, and the information is relevant to the working environment or policy under consideration. Nuffield sought to balance the costs to employee/employer and insuree/insurer, and went on to state that genetic screening would only be appropriate in the workplace when it would be too costly for employers to remove the environmental hazard, and genetic information could only be taken into account in insurance policies of a 'moderate size'. The council's 'light touch' on regulation and its vague definitions of costs now appear to have been inadequate, given the subsequent regulatory farce over insurance. The role of bodies such as the Nuffield in the policy network is too often a smokescreen for medico-scientific progress and when their conclusions are more critical they are too easy for governments and the market to ignored.

Professional codes of conduct

Another mushrooming form of genetics regulation is the professional code. Many of these codes concern the provision of genetic services, covering much of the technical detail about what tests to perform in what circumstances, and aiming for standardization of 'good practice'. Other codes comment on the wider ethical implications of genetics. Once more we can see these codes coalescing around a few key principles, based on informed consent and individual rights. This means that their conclusions tend to support all but the most ethically problematic practices. For example, the European Society of Human Genetics' recent inquiry into genetic information and testing in insurance (2000) stopped short of calling for a ban on the use of genetic information by insurance companies, and instead called for clear definitions and assessment procedures, collaboration between insurers and health care providers, and informed consent on the part of insurance applicants to the use of their test results, in situations where they were considered to be accurate and relevant. They are equally lax about the use of genetic information by employers, taking much the same line as the Nuffield Council seven years before them.

Professionals are not always so uncritical. A considerable number of well-placed geneticists reject gene patenting, and have been important lobbyists on this point. Geneticists also tend to be more critical of genetic testing of children, where their concern for informed consent means they view testing of children for late-onset disorders as particularly problematic, and tend not to countenance such procedures.[5]

But, more usually, professional codes and commentaries are narrow and unsatisfactory. For example, the American Society for Human Genetics (ASHG) regularly makes statements on genetics that are characteristic of the general trend in this field. ASHG emphasizes its commitment to rigorous research, informed choice and curing disease, covering topics such as eugenics and reproductive freedom, gene therapy and behavioural genetics. These statements tend to support developments in the fields of genetic testing, research and therapy, consigning eugenic abuse to the bad science of the past. Their central focus is the responsibility of the professional to provide unbiased information on the one hand, and to protect their patients on the other. Less criticism is given over to more controversial issues such as patenting and the rolling back of state health and welfare services for people who are poor or disabled. The ASHG even expressed support for the patenting of genes and genetic information with specific utility (although it opposed the patenting of DNA sequences with no demonstrated utility).[6] Geneticists are, in fact, supportive of much of the commercialization of genomics, as are governments. These alliances have resulted in a lax legislative approach to genetic research and development, and have even fostered genetic commodification and surveillance of entire populations, as we shall now go on to discuss.

The market network

We have already shown that geneticists have an important regulatory role through their position on various advisory bodies and commissions that guide international and national government policy and regulatory practices. And in our discussions of insurance we have shown how some geneticists, in alliance with actuaries, have played an important role in sanctioning the use of genetic information by insurance companies in the UK. Geneticists were, of course, instrumental in setting up many of the initial biotechnology companies with an interest in genomics, and have much to gain from the commercial exploitation of the field. But, as our discussion about Celera and the Human Genome Project (HGP) in Chapter 6 showed, the alliance between the public and private sectors in genomic research is often fraught.

This is particularly true where gene patenting is concerned. Despite the strong condemnation of gene patenting by the Wellcome Trust and leading British geneticists like Sir John Sulston of the Sanger Centre, the HGP's policy of open data has not staunched the flow of patent applications; indeed, it may even have intensified the race for patent approval, as private companies can utilise the public database for their own ends (as claimed in the war of words between representatives of the HGP and Celera). And geneticists have, for the most part, supported and even encouraged a limited framework of gene patenting where utility can be demonstrated. This means that geneticists tend to support the EU's patent directive of 1998 permitting the patenting of biological material isolated from its natural environment, so long at it is an invention that is novel, has industrial applicability and doesn't involve certain ethically problematic practices, including human cloning or germ-line engineering. HUGO and ASHG have also welcomed the position of the US Patent and Trademark Office (USPTO) where the gene, its function or its use can be patented, so long as its utility is 'specific, substantial and creditable'. Geneticists' reservations tend to be confined to DNA of unknown function or utility, which they view as raw data. But this type of boundary is difficult to sustain in practice. These rulings effectively sanction gene patenting on a massive scale, as the USPTO knows to its cost, given the thousands of patent applications by genomic companies that it is currently processing. Governments too have been supportive of a limited gene patenting framework, as we have previously discussed in Chapter 6. The regulation on patenting was devised hand in hand with the biotechnology and pharmaceutical industries, just as regimes of drug regulation have been devised by the state and the market in partnership.

Rather than viewing geneticists, the state and the market in isolation, we should think of them as being part of a fluid network of relations, where mutual interests are fundamental in shaping legislation and regulatory policies. This has resulted in lax regulation of gene patenting, despite the opposition of geneticists' associations like the American College of Medical Genetics, and funding bodies like the Wellcome Trust. A similar story can be told for the selective use of genetic information by insurance companies in the UK. Although the majority of geneticists oppose this practice, an influential grouping of actuaries and geneticists lobbied for and secured the practice. This group is also well represented on the regulatory body that oversees the use of test data. Even the recent HGC report on insurance was written in consultation with the ABI and the science minister, Lord Sainsbury. Although the ABI was less successful at influencing proceedings than previously, it remains an important player in this policy network.

But it is not just geneticists who have commercial associations and interests. We should also remember that various influential policy-making figures have commercial links to genetics. For example, Lord Sainsbury, the billionaire science minister, owned a company that controls a key gene currently used in the genetic modification process (the company was switched to a blind trust when he joined the government). Lord Winston, a Labour peer and IVF pioneer, recently obtained a patent on a technique that would allow researchers to genetically alter the human male germ-line cells that develop into sperm. Winston developed the technique in collaboration with researchers at the Cedars-Sinai Medical Center in Los Angeles and the California Institute of Technology in Pasadena, with funds from the American National Institutes of Health.[7]

An equally worrying trend in the contemporary regulation of genomics is the increasing collaboration between the state and the commercial sector over the collection, storage and exploitation of population genetic data. This is best exemplified by the Icelandic government's collaboration with deCode Genomics. In 1998 the Icelandic government passed the Icelandic Health Sector Database Act, and subsequently granted an exclusive licence on an electronic database of health information to deCode for twelve years at a time. The database will include information about all Icelanders who do not opt out of the scheme, and deCode will be able to add genetic and genealogical information to the database. As Andersen and Arnason note,

> deCode, through the act, has been permitted to break fundamental principles of scientific conduct: the requirement that research plans should be evaluated and approved by independent ethics committees before recruiting patients for studies. Without submitting a research plan, deCode convinced the Icelandic government that it should pass a law that avoided the necessity for review by the bioethics and data protection committees, the official regulatory bodies. While the government asked for the opinion of these committees after the bill was written, their recommendations on key issues, such as consent and exclusivity, were not followed.[8]

Despite repeated criticisms by the Icelandic Medical Association, the World Medical Association and other medical and scientific bodies, the Icelandic government continues to support the project. Critics have pointed out that although deCode and the Icelandic government claim the database is anonymous, centralizing the database of such a small population (275,000) and leaving it open to additions means that identification may be possible. And encryption can never guarantee full anonymity (someone still has to hold the encryption codes). The opt-out, rather than opt-in, strategy has also been heavily criticized, especially since it is quite difficult to achieve given the bureaucratic processes it involves, and once information is included in the database it cannot be withdrawn (around 20,000 people have opted out so far). But the government and deCode insist that it satisfies ethical standards and that the population ought to be altruistic, given the benefits that such research will bring. The Ministry of Health and Social Security of Iceland also considers that the database is acceptable from the perspective of international law.[9]

As we have noted, such a database is particularly valuable because it is thought that Iceland's population is homogenous, which makes it easier to trace mutations and understand the effects of the environment on disease. However, as research progresses, many critics have suggested that the population is far more heterogeneous than was first assumed. It is Iceland's store of data that is more fundamental. There are detailed medical records on the entire population, tissue samples of a large section of the population, and genealogical information on the majority of the population.[10] DeCode has filed patents and offers access to the database for a fee. It already has an exclusive deal with the pharmaceutical company Hoffman La Roche, allowing it access to the database to identify the genetic origins of twelve diseases. The hope is that the Icelandic population will benefit from the economic boost that this research will generate, and free drugs promised by Hoffman La Roche, but multinational firms are hardly bothered by national interests, given the global nature of pharmaceutical research and product development. Commerce is more likely to profit from this venture than the people of Iceland.

Although this is undoubtedly an extreme case of the state colluding with the market in the commodification of an entire population, it does involve practices that could be applied on a wider basis, as DNA registers and biomedical collections proliferate. In the UK the government and other advisory bodies, most recently the House of Lords Science and Technology Committee, have welcomed the Medical Research Council and Wellcome Trust's planned Population Biomedical Sample Collection which, although based firmly on the principle of informed consent and run by a non-profit-making organization, will still require collaboration with private capital to realize its potential in drug development and diagnostics. And informed consent is not a foolproof bulwark against exploitation, not least because people often do not know what they are consenting to and future uses cannot always be foreseen.

Other recent legislation concerning the confidentiality of medical information also presents a threat to patient autonomy. The Health and Social Care Act (2001) grants the Secretary of State for Health powers to pass regulations enforcing the processing of medical information for medical purposes in the public interest. Presented as a means by which the government can control the use of data by commercial companies, the Act effectively sanctions surveillance by government on a massive scale. As Simon Davies of the London School of Economics has pointed out, 'Individuals will lose their veto over the purposes for which their personal health information will be used . . . These powers will also allow data matching between the NHS, police, social services and Home Office and the Benefits Agency.'[11] Given the NHS's plans to create electronic health records for all patients, the biomedical and police forensic databases, and increasingly close ties between public services and the commercial market, it is not too far fetched to foresee this legislation being used to sanction commercial exploitation of population data on genetic disease. The medicalization of 'unhealthful behaviours', including criminality, may also be intensified by inter-agency and public–private collaborations such as these.

What these examples show is that, despite widespread condemnation by bioethicists, geneticists and other critics, the state will tend to favour commercial interests when they promise economic gain for the nation. The state will also use its powers of surveillance to over-ride individual rights in favour of what it characterizes as the public good, which in this era of global capital can mean the commodification of national resources like the population's DNA. The state shies away from stringent legislation to prevent abuse of genetic information, and relies on inadequate patent legislation to regulate the genomics sector. In Chapter 11 we go on to discuss how the market could be more effectively regulated, but before that we turn to consider public involvement in policy making about genetics.

Public involvement

Since the 1990s a coalition of scientists, politicians and government ministers have become increasingly concerned about public attitudes to new developments in genetics and associated biomedical ventures. Spurred by preoccupations about public fear and ignorance of genetics, a veritable industry of public education and consultation about genetics has emerged. It tends to be argued that, when presented with sufficient information, especially technical information about patterns of inheritance and probabilities, the public will appreciate the benefits of genetics and lose their irrational fears. Genetic knowledge will also protect us from a 'new eugenics', so the argument goes, by showing our common genetic heritage, and will increase tolerance, because genetics will show that people are not to blame for their anti-social behaviour or ill health, when these are located in their genes.

Although this 'deficit' model of public understanding of genetics has been roundly criticized, and public education initiatives have become more sophisticated as a result, an underlying scepticism about the public's capacity for reasoned input into genetic policy making remains. Technical knowledge is still valued above experiential knowledge. Yet pressure groups that are knowledgeable and critical are often marginalized in favour of the so-called general public, whose opinions are accessed through a range of surveys and opinion polls that are now routinely conducted by government agencies and funding bodies like the Wellcome Trust. As Davison and colleagues have noted, interest groups are seen as unduly biased and atypical minorities, so they tend to be excluded, or, if included, treated as special, unusual cases. Survey results can thus become a substitute for proper public debate, by ignoring or 'exoticizing' special interest groups.[12]

Davison and colleagues continue that, as biotechnology moves closer to the market, survey respondents are increasingly being treated as consumers, not citizens. Questions are typically closed and there is no room for spontaneous input, or critical commentary, on the style of questions. Respondents are asked to weigh up the pros and cons of genetics. 'Science' tends to be narrowly defined, as neutral and objective, with overwhelmingly positive applications. It is often presented as easy to control with proper regulation. Scientists are frequently presented as responsible professionals, with the public good as their principal motivator, not commercial profit. When commerce is discussed (usually in relation to food production) the emphasis is often upon science providing consumers with more and better choices. Respondents tend to be led down a particular route of response that maximizes support and minimizes criticism of genetics. For example, 'Would you allow your child to have gene therapy in order to treat a genetic disease?' is asked, rather than a question about people's views on the commercial environment in which technologies such as these are being developed.

The majority 'public opinion' then becomes an entity in its own right – an attitude, not a behaviour, as Brian Wynne has argued.[13] Little or no attention is paid to why the public know what they know (other than their level of knowledge about scientific facts), or about what they might like to know. Public opinion statistics are then mobilized in policy-making discussions. When the statistics are supportive this is used to counter criticism and underline scientists' democratic mandate. When support is less apparent, the media are often criticized for misrepresentation, and better education is advocated. Rarely do negative public opinion poll results have an effect on policy. At worst, surveys on genetics have little to do with democracy and empowerment of the public, and are closely associated with 'manufacturing consent', stifling dissent and promoting the interests of commerce and industry. As Davison and colleagues note, 'Polling has become a tool not for engaging "the public" in the business of public life, but for the creation of a simulacrum of politics.'[14]

Public consultation processes also remain flawed, despite their stated aims of openness and accountability. In the UK, the HGC and associated bodies have engaged in these exercises for some time, for example through issuing documents listing a set of questions that respondents can then address in written responses to the commission. The commission also calls witnesses to public meetings, where they answer questions. Not surprisingly, it is experts who dominate these sessions, asking and answering most of the questions. Rarely do ordinary members of the public submit their views. An example of the flaws in consultation is provided by the ACGT/HFEA consultation on pre-implantation genetic diagnosis (PGD) in 2000. This took place long after PGD had been developed at the Hammersmith. The consultation was cursory. At the time of writing, sixteen months after the deadline for submissions, no results have been published.

Organizations like the Genetics Interest Group (GIG) and other patients' groups are, of course, involved in these consultation processes. But these organizations have their own priorities, and links with science and industry. For example, when GIG director Alistair Kent recently spoke at a conference entitled 'Capitalising on Genetic Variation' (organized by the pharmaceutical industry) his talk was titled: 'Harnessing the power of patient groups to influence government policy on pharmacogenetically developed drugs to ensure that you stay abreast of public feeling'. Patients' groups like GIG are certainly influential in policy making, and their views are undoubtedly important. But they are not a substitute for proper public involvement, nor do they represent the views of people with genetic disorders who are less enamoured with scientific progress and commercial gain.

Although we are critical of contemporary forms of public consultation about genetics, we do recognize that they are a valuable route towards more sustained, critical and interactive methods of involving the public in policy making in this area; methods that we will discuss further shortly. We will also discuss ways in which bioethics could be developed to provide a more critical commentary on genetics, and how we can promote regulation and legislation that would prevent the rise of a new eugenics. But we are far more sceptical about the benefits of links between genetics, the state and the genomics market, as outlined in the previous section. Without a critical distance from the interests of commerce, the state is not well placed to protect the people it is supposed to represent, as the

Icelandic experience so graphically illustrates. As representative democracy ossifies, we must look to community participation and activism that cuts across global and national, corporate, professional and political interests, and challenges eugenics from below. We explore what this might mean in the final chapter.

11
Conclusion

In the public discourse of geneticists, China is usually the exception that proves their rule that nowadays we have no reason to worry about eugenics. But are the Chinese policies on disability and genetics so different from those of the industrialized North? The Maternal and Infant Health Care Law was passed in China in 1994, and came into effect the following year. Although the original draft of the law provoked widespread international condemnation, and was amended to remove terms like 'inferior' and 'eugenic' and to make sterilization and abortion 'voluntary' rather than 'obligatory', the law that was passed insists on genetic counselling if either partner is disabled, and abortion if a pregnancy is affected by 'serious hereditary diseases' or 'relevant medical disorders', including AIDS, venereal disease, leprosy, congenital impairments, schizophrenia and conditions that prevent independent living, or can be inherited by the next generation. Disabled people can marry and have children, as long as they will not be affected by disability, and abortion is advised if impairment is detected in a foetus. The strong government message is that impairment is undesirable and unnatural and should be prevented if possible. Although there are no explicit laws like this in the industrialized North, many of these values are implicit, and sometimes even explicit, in genetic counselling sessions and public health rationales for genetic screening programmes, as we have demonstrated throughout this book.

Chinese attitudes to disabled people are also similar to those in the North. Emma Stone notes that the situation for China's 51 million disabled people has vastly improved in recent years, as a result of the Law on the Protection of Disabled Persons (1990), drafted by the Chinese Disabled Persons' Federation. During the 1980s, China adopted international approaches to disability, promoted by the UN World Programme of Action Concerning Disabled Persons, and other international programmes that emphasize integration, rehabilitation and prevention. In the 1980s, under Deng Xiaoping, there was a national survey of the disabled population, and concerted efforts were made to find them work and improve their quality of life, under the slogan 'I serve the disabled and the disabled serve society.' The 1990 law ensures civil rights, integration and participation for disabled people.[1] As Stone argues, China emulated the rest of the world: 'Chinese policy-makers have done no more and no less than their counterparts throughout the industrialised North, except that they made the mistake of using language no longer *au fait*. Eugenics is out; maternal and infant health care is in.'[2]

Stone's analysis suggests that we should be wary of exoticizing Chinese eugenics as so very different from the practices of the North. Her discussion also shows that a policy of eliminating disability through reproductive interventions can sit happily with social policies designed to increase the civil rights of people already living with disabilities. This is because the two policies are not as different as they first appear. Both are concerned with maximizing people's social contribution, whether this involves the avoidance of a disabled child or overcoming their disability through productive labour. In a sense, civil rights are a byproduct of this emphasis on people's social worth. Disabled people's civil rights therefore remain limited, especially when it comes to reproductive choice. Although our policies of discrimination against disabled people in the North are far less overt, we can see traces of these attitudes and approaches in the way health and welfare services are organized for disabled people. The attitudes and relationships that form the basis of the way contemporary society approaches disability and genetics come from our eugenic heritage. So what are the keystones of this legacy?

Looking back

There are four main similarities between genetic politics in the past and the present that we wish to highlight here. First, as Stone comments, today, as in the past, we continue to hold contradictory attitudes towards disabled people, largely based on a mixture of fear, suspicion and pity. These attitudes profoundly shape the problems addressed by genetic research and the modes of intervention developed to resolve them. In both the eras of mainline eugenics and genomics the categories of 'genetic disease' expanded. There has always been a focus on the physically and mentally disabled, throughout the history of eugenics and genetics. Other socially stigmatized groups, such as people who are mentally ill, addicts or criminals, or children with behavioural difficulties, are also focused upon in the era of mainline eugenics and in today's genomics. The genetic gaze has extended still further, to take in a whole range of common diseases, such as cancer and heart disease. And, although the crude racism of the past has been rejected, racial differences in people's propensity to disease and social deviance continue to be of interest.

Contemporary approaches to people with these so-called genetic diseases and disorders are also similar to those of the past, to the extent that their conditions are considered to be in need of treatment, and to result from their heredity, rather than their environment. This requires particular kinds of treatment, based upon genetic testing, to provide a diagnosis. What is striking about the genetic advances of the modern era, is that the bulk of interventions that take place tend to concentrate, now as in the past, on reproductive interventions. This is not to deny that there is a huge investment in developing genetic treatments, or to suggest that prenatal testing is currently available for multifactorial conditions or minor disorders. But, so far, reproductive interventions far outweigh the possibilities for successful genetic treatments, let alone cures.

Although overt coercion to participate in genetic testing is far less common in today's neoliberal democracies, there are many subtle and not-so-subtle ways in which people are pressurized to comply with genetic testing, particularly in screening programmes. There is a widespread view amongst clinicians, scientists and policy-makers, that the birth of a disabled child is a tragedy best avoided. Just as in the past, professionals are making decisions about what kinds of people ought to be born, and these decisions have a profound effect on people undergoing genetic diagnosis and making the ultimate choice about whether or not to continue with their pregnancies. More generally, in society at large, disabled people face stigma, poverty and poor health and welfare provision. Although their situation is obviously improved from that of the past, discrimination continues to affect their lives, and those of their families.

Second, throughout the history of eugenics and genetics, professionals have held an inordinate amount of power and control over what genetic research gets conducted; how genetics is applied in the clinic and beyond in the wider community; and how genetic research and services are regulated. We do not wish to draw any simple parallels between the totalitarianism of Nazi Germany, the welfare states of Scandinavia, the paternalism and bigotries of the British and American states at the height of mainline eugenics, and the current vogue of neoliberalism, as there are clearly many differences in the ways in which genetic choices are offered and enacted in these different contexts and eras. But professionals remain at the heart of policy making about genetics today, as in the past. Their interest in the expansion of research and services drives much of policy and practice in this area. By and large, other key players in policy discussions, such as professional bioethicists, are also too sanguine about the risks and problems associated with increasing geneticization and technological expansion. Alongside their genetics allies, they continue to make pronouncements and judgements about the good of society, and to construct policies to manage genetics for these ends. The ideal of individual, patient choice may now be paramount, but professional control remains fundamental in the laboratory, the clinic and the policy-making arena.

With this professional dominance come several crucial modes of understanding and practising science and technology, which can also be traced to the early days of genetics and eugenics. The third commonality between the past and the present that we wish to highlight here is the technocratic ideal, where knowledge is set apart from technology, seemingly objective and neutral to be wisely applied, rather than challenged in its own terms. This framing of science and technology remains crucial to genomic policy making and professional rhetoric about genetic progress, as we go on to discuss shortly. Policy discussions still tend to focus almost exclusively on the social implications of genetic knowledge and technologies, as if the knowledge and technology were somehow inevitable and immune to social critique in their own right. Yet the history and present of genetics shows that the content of science and its implications cannot be so easily separated.

Fourth, eugenics and genomics across the globe also share one apparently over-arching guiding principle – progress. The grand schemes of the past to eliminate disease and suffering in the interests of social progress chime with the contemporary rhetoric of disease prevention in discussions about the Human Genome Project and associated genetic services. But when critics point to the dangers of progress down certain paths, they are dismissed as fearful and ignorant. Scientists play their trump card of expert knowledge to impose their version of how science progresses along ethically acceptable lines. Just as in the past, when critics of the new genetics or other areas of scientific research warned of future developments, advocates of science suggest that this is scaremongering. Terms such as 'designer babies' and 'genetic underclass' are rejected as being unfeasible. The various independent or state-sponsored bodies which exist to reassure the public that state and science are being responsible do not tend to evaluate things that are not possible at that stage of research. As Barbara Katz Rothman argues, 'The scientists quickly speak up: that isn't possible, they reassure us, you don't understand the genetics involved. Five years later, of course, that *is* possible, and then it is too late to decide whether or not to do it: we wake up to find it done.'[3]

In the absence of explicit regulation, scientists can be given free rein to develop novel procedures, such as pre-implantation genetic diagnosis or somatic nuclear replacement (cloning). Later, a commission may get around to discussing the issue, and will conclude that as the research or practice is already taking place, it is impossible to turn back the clock and prevent it. In this way, progress along a certain path appears inevitable, but it is the structures of power and decision making that make it so, not the knowledge itself.

In the past and the present, we can see that the reality of progress in policy making is that there tends to be a move, by slow degrees, into a situation that would have been unacceptable to the public or to parliamentarians if presented to them in full at the outset. A good example of this is embryo research regulation in the UK. Effective lobbying by scientists, based on the promise of cures for rare diseases, led to the most liberal embryo research regime in the world, arising from the 1990 Human Fertilisation and Embryology Act. Ten years later, the grounds for embryo experimentation have been extended to allow research on the therapeutic properties of embryonic stem cells and therapeutic cloning. Opponents of this move are told that there is no legal distinction between this research and the existing permission granted in 1990. Yet, as the research develops the technology of somatic cell nuclear transfer, we are moving closer to the acceptance of reproductive cloning, despite the claims to the contrary. Many doctors and scientists believe that reproductive cloning will take place within the next ten years. As Jonathan Glover has commented in a different context, 'By easy stages we could move to a world which none of us would choose if we could see it as a whole from the start.'[4]

Turning from research to clinical practice, a similar incrementalism can also be observed. Doctors engage in 'shroud waving' in specific clinical cases as well as in the general advocacy of medical research. Both are ways of appealing to our sympathy for those affected by difficult situations – infertility or impairment or illness – and transferring this sympathy into the acceptance of blurred ethical boundaries or utilitarian justifications for new morally suspect processes. New technologies or processes are introduced in one-off cases as the solution to a heart-rending problem. In general, the history of medical technologies shows that they can soon become generalized and applied to a much bigger group of patients than was ever envisaged.

This means that individual reproductive choice could lead to a designer baby future, as outlined by the embryologist Lee Silver in his book *Remaking Eden*. He argues that increasing technological powers – gene chips for diagnosis, polymerase chain reaction for amplifying DNA, cloning to create additional embryos – plus a market system based on the rhetoric of individual choice could lead to selection of embryos on the grounds of non-pathological characteristics such as intelligence, physical abilities or temperament. Clearly none of these things is straightforwardly genetically determined. But genes of small effect undoubtedly play a role in many illnesses and behaviours, and it is not too far-fetched to imagine that manipulation will be desired by many ambitious parents who currently invest in private education, extra language or tennis coaching, and cosmetic surgery and orthodontics for their families.

The definition and treatment of the so-called genetically diseased, the privileging of professional authority, the technocratic ideal and the fetish of progress create many problems in the ways in which our society thinks about genetics, regulates genetics and practises genetics, both in the past and in the present. This means that eugenics can be an emergent property of the regulatory system as well as the more general nexus of cultural values and social relationships in research and services concerned with disability and genetics in contemporary society. Contemporary policies focus upon countering the danger of overt eugenics, like state-sponsored oppression or ethically dubious research such as reproductive cloning, but they are ineffective at stemming eugenic outcomes such as professional and wider societal pressures to comply with genetic screening and abortion, discrimination by insurance companies and employers, and even possibly reproductive cloning, via therapeutic cloning. There are no robust boundaries to limit the application of biotechnical solutions to social problems: for example, we believe that the technologies that are currently used mainly for therapeutic purposes will increasingly be used for purposes of enhancement. And the nexus of relationships between professionals, the state and the market fuels the potential for a commercialized eugenics, which will exacerbate inequalities in wealth and status. As Barbara Katz Rothman suggests, 'In the hands of the market, the "book of life" becomes a catalog.'[5]

To reduce the potential for eugenics, we need to think differently about genetic policy making and practice, and to develop a more realistic appraisal of science and technology where it is understood in its wider social context. We also need to open up policy making to other interested parties, and challenge professional dominance of decision making. On a more philosophical note, our attitudes to choice, life and disability also require rethinking. We now explore what alternatives we have open to us. What principles, practices and policies should underpin the development of genetic science to avoid a negative future, and to foster a just and ethical relationship between science and society?

Thinking hard

If there is truth in our warning about the future, then it behoves us to consider urgently whether there is a better way of thinking about humanity. For a starting point, we could turn to the words of Archbishop, and former scientist, John Habgood, in his 1995 Heslington Lecture:

> First, human beings are more than their genes. Genes are only a set of instructions. We are more than a set of instructions. Second rule: remember the valuable diversity of human nature. Third rule: look for justice in the dealings of human beings with one another, and for fairness in the use of resources. Fourth rule: respect privacy and autonomy. Fifth rule: accept the presumption that disease should be cured when it is possible to do so. And sixth rule: be very suspicious about improving human nature; and be even more suspicious of those who think they know what improvement should be made.[6]

Although we share the Archbishop's stress on diversity, justice and fairness, and his rejection of improvement to human nature, his solution remains inadequate. The Archbishop's scientific roots are showing when he emphasizes curing disease and respecting autonomy. We need to develop a different approach to disease and disability and to be wary of appeals to individual choice.

Disability and difference should be respected, not eliminated. While we agree that parents should be able to avoid the suffering associated with some extreme genetic conditions, most genetic conditions are not of this order. Disabled people have argued that the main problems of disability are social, not genetic. We should remove the environmental and economic barriers that disable people, not remove people who have impairments. As the feminist Meg Stacey argues,

> Tidying away some heritable diseases will not make the society tidy, nor will it eliminate suffering. Has the time come perhaps when it is necessary to revise the scientific goal to one which would work with nature rather than attempting to beat it? Inevitably we shall be born and die. That is how the human organism is. Inevitably we shall become ill and some of us will be disabled. Medicine would have much to offer in such a co-operative enterprise.[7]

This approach is endorsed by some biologists too: 'Genetic imperfection is an unavoidable characteristic of human hereditary processes; it is part of what makes us human.'[8] That is, evolution depends on diversity, as Limoges argues: 'After all, it is genetic "errors" that made us a biological species: we humans are integrated aggregates of such "errors".'[9]

This alternative ethic of care and compassion for disability and difference, which values diversity and tolerates the mixed fortunes and complex relationships of dependency that frame our lives, suggests a very different path for genetic medicine. We are not naïve enough to assume that this ethic can be easily transplanted into modern genomics, and we recognize that many of the values of stigma and ignorance that shape its current form are prevalent in society at large. But this does not mean that we should not tap into people's everyday ethics of care and seek to articulate that in public discussions and policy making about genetics, in order to foster a more humane form of genetic medicine, and to undermine the drivers towards a eugenic future.

We also need to think differently about individuals' choices, seeing them as part of a wider social context in terms of how they are expressed, and the consequences they might have. Kavka's notion of upside risks helps us to understand this. In some situations an individual might benefit from pursuing a particular strategy, but social problems arise if everyone follows the same approach. An obvious example would be the use of motor cars: for each individual, it makes sense, but if all of us drive, we end up with traffic jams and global pollution. Kavka gives various examples of the ways in which biotechnology might lead to upside risks. One is a collective imbalance in the population caused by individual reproductive decisions: for example, in certain societies, the desire for a male child has led to an alteration of the sex ratio. Another is the increased social inequality that would result from the scenario outlined by Silver above: IVF and embryo biopsy are expensive, and will only be available to the rich. Enhancing the quality of children will further disadvantage lower socio-economic groups. Third, collective attitudes to disability will be influenced if people exercise their individual choice to avoid the birth of disabled children, because toleration of difference and abnormality will be reduced. We continue to be told that the abortion of disabled foetuses says nothing about the care of people already living with disabilities. But if disability is seen as a problem that should be avoided prenatally, then views of disabled people change for the worse, and services for disabled people suffer. 'Dependent' disabled people are still unwelcome because our society stresses individual competition and market solutions: if our communities valued and supported people with impairments such as learning difficulties, then disability would not be seen as such a problem. Finally, an overemphasis on scientific and technical solutions may lead to individuals having an increased sense of responsibility, as they have to make more and more choices about how to have families and run their lives. Kavka argues that this might lead to existential dread, and a paralysis of choice.[10]

This means that we need to promote a different understanding of choice, where individuals' choices are seen as intrinsically shaped by the society of which they are a part, and to have consequences beyond their immediate family. People should be able to choose to have a disabled child, and resources must be provided to allow them to do so. Not all individual choices to abort are acceptable, and boundaries must be set in place to prevent the slippage into screening for more minor impairments. In short, liberty should not be confused with licence, and it should be tempered with a respect for equality.

Policy pragmatics

In addition to these alternative philosophies of life and choice, there are several more practical, concrete steps that we could take to regulate genomics and prevent eugenics. Despite our scepticism about the regulatory process, there is room for improvement in both the mechanisms and outcomes of contemporary legislation concerning genetics. It seems obvious which policies need to change, but let's be clear nonetheless. We need more robust and effective regulation around privacy and discrimination based on genetic information. We need regulation to restrict patenting much more forcibly, at the international and national levels. We need to step back from implementing further genetic screening programmes in the National Health Service, and to reconsider those which are currently on offer. The private sector must be controlled more effectively, and prevented from dictating policy in the health service, and in drug regulation and development. The commercial market for genetic tests and screening services ought to be staunched. We believe that prenatal tests for minor genetic disorders or behavioural characteristics should not be developed, and that if such information becomes available indirectly then it should be ignored. Research into behavioural genetics should be stopped or, at the very least, seriously curtailed.

In providing this 'wish list' we open ourselves up to charges of naïvety and stubborn retrenchment. But we think our arguments throughout this book have demonstrated that it is our critics who are naïve and stubborn in their commitment to progress at all costs. Our assessment of genetic science and technology demonstrates that it is a thoroughly social process, therefore it is open to, not immune from, social change. Cultural values can change, just as social relationships can change, to foster a different science of genetics and a different way of controlling its development and implications. We accept that the types of change we envisage are a long way off, but this does not mean they are futile. On a more pragmatic note, we can see several routes by which change can be fostered, albeit slowly and with much resistance from the powers that be.

Let us start by thinking about science, technology and progress. We need to challenge the idea that knowledge and technology are immune from social critique, or indeed influence. Instead, we need to recognize that social values are embedded in the fabric of our knowledge and our technologies. Once we have recognized this, we can proceed to think about which values we want to see our knowledge and technology reflect. This means that we have to consider what type of research is conducted and what technologies are developed and implemented in our name. We need to develop techniques for evaluating the potential social implications of particular forms of knowledge and technology before they are set in motion, not after the event. We need to see the commercial market as the product of our collective labours (and, increasingly, our DNA), which cannot simply be controlled through our consumption, but must also be controlled by government. And we need to see the connections between and across seemingly disconnected technical and knowledge paths, noting how practices can slip beyond their original remit, to include more tests or more populations subject to screening, for example. This is not a call for policy-makers to develop some sort of sixth sense so that they can know the future. Instead it is a call for caution and increased awareness of the connections between techniques and populations that have been made in the past, and of how knowledge and technology evolves in the market place.

We also need to debunk the notion of technological inevitability. As Donald MacKenzie has pointed out in his book *Inventing Accuracy*,

> Outside of the human, intellectual, and material network that give them life and force, technologies cease to exist. We cannot reverse the invention of the motor car, perhaps, but imagine a world in which there were no car factories, no gasoline, no roads, where no one alive had ever driven, and where there was satisfaction with whatever alternative form of transportation existed. The libraries might still contain pictures of automobiles and texts on motor mechanics, but there would be a sense in which that was a world in which the motor car had been uninvented.[11]

Just as motor cars, or even nuclear missiles, need not be inevitable, designer babies or a genetic underclass are not inevitable, if we challenge the values and practices that can lead us to this future.

Greater public involvement in decision making, and less reliance on professional and industry experts and lobbyists, might be one way to foster these alternatives. We believe that the dangers of eugenics can be forestalled, in part, by vibrant, contradictory and pluralistic debate and discussion in the wider community, which could then be fed into policy making, in an obvious and direct manner. Expert opinions still need to be voiced, but in a forum where alternative perspectives based on people's experiences, for example of illness and disability, are also heard. As we said earlier, we need to provide public arenas to allow people to *think* about these issues, not just to choose or decide on the topic of the day. We need to foster a wide range of expertise, and challenge prejudice and ignorance, held by professionals as well as publics. This means promoting an alternative ethic of care, the social model of disability, as well as a more contextual understanding of choice, science and technology. As we have already argued, we believe that these understandings come from people's everyday experiences, but that this understanding needs to be nurtured to undermine the current tendency to privilege technical expertise and commercial hype.

Although we have been highly critical of bioethics, we would also like to stress that bioethics from the ground up, based on careful consideration of how morality is enacted in society – from the boardroom, to the clinic, to the high street – instead of normative prescriptions about choice and progress, would also be essential to more sophisticated policy making. We would like to think that social researchers could work with their bioethical colleagues in this project, but we remain cautious about simply assuming the role of expert about publics, instead of truly involving publics in decision making about genetic research, services and implications.

In addition to these 'legitimate' solutions there are, of course, other smaller-scale subversive routes that could be pursued to undermine contemporary forms of eugenics. We have already mentioned patients' and professionals' strategies for protecting people from genetic discrimination: from not taking the test, to testing once insurance has been arranged, to reinterpreting the meaning of genetic test results in the wider context of an individual's or a family's circumstances. Patients' groups and critical professionals have also formed valuable alliances to challenge patenting, even at times taking out their own patents on genes or genetic procedures and then refusing to enforce them in order to foster research and better genetic tests. These groups can also be important in stemming the genetic determinism in simplistic media accounts, by presenting their own experiences and perspectives.

On a more global scale there is much to be learned from activists involved in protesting against genetically modified foods, who have formed valuable alliances across the North–South divide. Similarly, protests against commercialization and commodification by transnational corporations, and successful challenges to large drug companies' patents on life-saving drugs that are too expensive for developing countries, point the way to global resistance to genetic patenting and discrimination. And the growing pressure for accountable and democratic decision making in challenge to the mantra of free trade also has implications for genetic services and treaties at the international level. Genomics demands both global and local monitoring and controls through democratic means. Otherwise global eugenics will flourish once more.

Notes

Chapter 1 Introduction

1. Paul, 1992: 665.
2. Shakespeare, 1999.
3. Caplan, 1994: 41.
4. Clarke, 1991.
5. Lenaghan, 1998: 48.
6. Rogers, 1999.
7. Kerr *et al.*, 1998c.
8. Wald *et al.*, 1992.
9. Glover, 1999: 116.
10. Glover, 1984: 31.
11. Paul, 1992: 669.
12. Duster, 1990.
13. Kitcher, 1996.
14. Searle, 1997.

Chapter 2 The rise of eugenics in the UK and the USA

1. MacKenzie, 1976.
2. Rosenberg, 1997.
3. Cravens, 1978: 3; noted in Paul, 1998a: 10.
4. Lowe, 1979: 304.
5. Farrall, 1970.
6. Farrall, 1970: 38.
7. Kevles, 1995: 60.
8. Paul, 1998b: 14.
9. Soloway, 1997: 54.
10. Kevles, 1995: 63.
11. Kevles, 1995: 67; quoting Goodhue, 1913: 155.
12. Allen, 1983.
13. Pernick, 1997.
14. Kevles, 1995: 62.
15. Allen, 1983: 120.
16. Trombley, 1988: 139.
17. Prichard, 1963: 133.
18. Prichard, 1963: 188.
19. Potts and Fido, 1991: 11.
20. Quoted in Paul, 1998a: 82.

Chapter 3   Nazi racial science

1. Friedlander, 1995: 7.
2. Burleigh, 1994.
3. Friedlander, 1995: 30ff.
4. Gallagher, 1995: 23.
5. Friedlander, 1995: 62.
6. Burleigh, 1994: 112.
7. Gallagher, 1995: 31.
8. Friedlander, 1995: 80.
9. Friedlander, 1995: 61.
10. Friedlander, 1995: 45.
11. Gallagher, 1995: 103.
12. Friedlander, 1995: 284.
13. Gallagher, 1995: xv.
14. Gallagher, 1995: xv.
15. Gallagher, 1995: 171.
16. Burleigh, 1994: 105.
17. Gallagher, 1995: 115.
18. Friedlander, 1995: 108.
19. Gallagher, 1995: 201.
20. Friedlander, 1995: 188.
21. Friedlander, 1995: 295.
22. Burleigh, 1994: 97.

Chapter 4   Eugenics in democratic societies

1. Unpublished paper.
2. Quoted in Broberg and Tydén, 1996: 85.
3. Myrdal, 1968: 215.
4. Hansen, 1996: 20.
5. Hansen, 1996: 29.
6. Adapted from T. Kemp, *Arvehygiejne, Københavns Årsskrift* (Copenhagen: Københavns Universitet, 1951), p. 45.
7. Hietala, 1996.
8. See Adams, 1990; Drouard, 1998; Graham, 1977, 1981; Maier, 1936; Schneider, 1990.
9. Broberg and Tydén, 1996: 136.

Chapter 5   Reform eugenics from the 1930s to the 1970s

1. Mazumdar, 1992: 258.
2. Watt, 1998: 138.
3. Gudding, 1996.
4. Paul, 1998b: 137.
5. Resta, 1997; quoted in Petersen, 1999.
6. Sutton, 1967: 22.
7. Emery, 1968.

8.   Gudding, 1996.
9.   Martin, 1999.
10. Emery, 1968.
11. Emery, 1968.
12. Cowan, 1994.
13. Paul, 1998a: 129.
14. McKusick, 1970: 27.
15. Martin and Hoehn, 1974: 403.
16. Paul, 1998b: 167.
17. Paul, 1998b: 174; referring to Edelson, forthcoming.
18. Paul, 1998b: 181.
19. Kevles, 1995: 256.
20. Thomson, 1999: 294.
21. Trombley, 1988: 178.
22. Trombley, 1988: 202.
23. Trombley, 1988: 206.
24. Trombley, 1988: 203.
25. Pfeiffer, 1994: 495.
26. Trombley, 1988: 176–7.
27. Kaye, 1997: 78; discussing Handler, 1970.
28. Gudding, 1996.
29. Gieryn and Figert, 1986.
30. Paul, 1998a: 85.
31. Paul, 1998a: 86.

Chapter 6   The rise of the new genetics

1.   Wright, 1986.
2.   Wright, 1986: 355.
3.   Krimsky, 1982.
4.   Martin, 1999: 522–3.
5.   Mulkay, 1997: 68.
6.   Cook-Deegan, 1994: 42.
7.   Bodmer quoted in Lewontin, 1991: 75.
8.   http://www.ornl.gov/hgmis/home.html.
9.   Malakoff and Service, 2001.
10. Gillis, 2000a.
11. Gillis, 2000b.
12. Smaglik, 2000.
13. Bobrow and Thomas, 2001.
14. Dobson, 2000.
15. Wolf *et al.*, 2000.
16. Marteau and Croyle, 1998: 694.
17. British Society for Human Genetics, 1999. See
     http://www.bham.ac.uk/BSHG/raredis.htm.
18. Clayton, 1999: 112.
19. Lehrman, www.dnaprofiles.org/about/pgm/topic.html.
20. McGuffin *et al.*, 2001.

21. Fraser, 1995: 2.
22. Lind in Fraser, 1995: 176.
23. Macdonald, 1997: 632.
24. Pfeiffer, 1994.

Chapter 7   Genetics as culture

1. Lippman, 1992a.
2. Nelkin and Lindee, 1995: 57.
3. Nelkin and Lindee, 1995: 2.
4. Van Dijck, 1998: 183.
5. Van Dijck, 1998: 130.
6. Watson, 1997: 624.
7. Ryan, 1999: 127.
8. Van Dijck, 1998: 12.
9. Fujimura, 1988.
10. Van Dijck, 1995: 10.
11. Mulkay, 1997: 72.
12. Lippman, 1992b.
13. Conrad, 1999.
14. Henderson and Kitzinger, 1999.
15. Rothman, 1998: 23.
16. Alper and Beckwith, 1994.
17. Kaplan, 2000.
18. Murray, 2000: 30.
19. Nelkin and Lindee, 1995: 101.
20. Bateson and Martin, 1999: 66.
21. Bateson and Martin, 1999: 59.
22. Bateson and Martin, 1999: 60.
23. Skuse *et al.*, 1997.
24. Owen and Cardno, 1999: 13.
25. Owen and Cardno, 1993: 14.
26. Rose and Rose, 2000.
27. Condit, 1999.
28. Kerr *et al.*, 1998a and 1998b.
29. Novas and Rose, 2000.

Chapter 8   Choice in social context

1. Van Dijck, 1998: 97.
2. Taylor, 1998.
3. Clarke, 1994: 16ff.
4. Britton and Knox, 1991.
5. Lippman and Wilfond, 1992.
6. Bailey, 1996: 164.
7. Green, 1994.
8. Marteau *et al.*, 1994; Marteau *et al.*, 1993.
9. Farrant, 1985.

10. Green, 1995.
11. Toy, 2000.
12. Kerr *et al.*, 1996: 21.
13. Lukes, 1974: 23.
14. Porter and Macintyre, 1984.
15. Marteau *et al.*, 1988.
16. Green and Statham, 1996: 143.
17. Rothman, 1998: 120.
18. Rothman, 1998: 192.
19. Rothman, 1988: 101.
20. Nelkin and Lindee, 1995: 166.
21. House of Commons Science and Technology Committee, 1995.
22. Hallowell, 1999.
23. Rothman, 1988.
24. Wexler, 1970.
25. Marteau and Richards, 1996.
26. Marteau and Richards, 1996.
27. Rothman, 1998: 212.
28. Rothman, 1988: 180.
29. Clarke and Flinter, 1996; Davis, 2001.
30. Wolbring, personal communication.
31. Asch and Geller, 1996.
32. Hubbard, 1997: 187.
33. Dworkin, 1993.

Chapter 9   The consequences of choice

1.   http://www.gene-watch.org/programs/TakingLiberties.html.
2.   Marteau and Drake, 1995.
3.   Glannon, 1998.
4.   Harris, 1998.
5.   Buchanan *et al.*, 2000.
6.   Beck-Gernsheim, 1990: 455.
7.   Beck-Gernsheim, 1990: 459.
8.   Hubbard, 1997: 199.
9.   Harper and Clarke, 1997.
10. Pokorski, 1994: 106.
11. Hubbard and Wald, 1993: 142.
12. Harper in Harper and Clarke, 1997.
13. Curtis *et al.*, 1997.
14. Lenaghan, 1998.
15. Lenaghan, 1998: 109.
16. Knoppers, 1999.
17. Burn quoted in Lenghan, 1998: 101.
18. Duster and Beeson, 2001.
19. NOP poll quoted in Lenaghan, 1998: 101.
20. Peterson and Lupton, 1996.
21. Hallowell, 1999.

22. Berger, 1999.
23. Medical Research Council, 2000.
24. Nelkin and Andrews, 1999: 203.
25. Concar, 2001a.
26. Concar, 2001b.
27. Rose, 2000.
28. DeGrandpre, 2000.
29. Rose, 2000: 24.

Chapter 10　Regulating genetics

1. Jonsen, 1998.
2. Jonsen, 1988: 182.
3. Caplan *et al.*, 1999: 1284.
4. Anon., 1999.
5. Clinical Genetics Society Working Party, 1994.
6. American Society of Human Genetics, 1991.
7. Rogers, 2000.
8. Andersen and Arnason, 1999: 1565.
9. Chadwick, 1999.
10. Berger, 1999.
11. Anon., 2001.
12. Davison *et al.*, 1997.
13. Wynne, 1995.
14. Davison *et al.*, 1997: 330.

Chapter 11　Conclusion

1. Stone, 1996.
2. Stone, 1996: 477.
3. Rothman, 1998: 37.
4. Glover 1984: 14.
5. Rothman 1998: 218.
6. Reiss and Straughan, 1996: 221.
7. Stacey, 1996: 346.
8. Suzuki and Knudtson, 1989: 205.
9. Limoges, 1994: 124.
10. Kavka, 1994.
11. MacKenzie, 1990: 426.

Bibliography

Abberley, P. (1987) 'The concept of oppression and the development of a social theory of disability', *Disability, Handicap and Society*, 2, 1, pp. 5–21.

Adams, M. B. (1990) *The Wellborn Science: Eugenics in Germany, France, Brazil and Russia*, New York: Oxford University Press.

Allen, G. (1983) 'The misuse of biological hierarchies: the American eugenics movement, 1900–1940', *History and Philosophy of the Life Sciences*, 5, 2, pp. 105–28.

Alper, J. S. and Beckwith, J. (1994) 'Genetic fatalism and social policy: the implications of behavior genetic research', *Yale Journal of Biology and Medicine*, 66, pp. 511–24.

American Society of Human Genetics (Human Genome Committee) (1991) Untitled [Letter], 254, 5039, pp. 1710–12.

Andersen, B. and Arnason, E. (1999) 'Iceland's database is ethically questionable', *British Medical Journal*, 318, p. 1565.

Anon. (1999) 'WHO steps closer to its responsibilities', *Nature*, 398, p. 175.

Anon. (2001) 'Trust me I'm a Health Minister', www.kablenet.com, 13 March.

Appleyard, B. (1999) *Brave New Worlds: Staying human in the genetic future*, London: HarperCollins.

Asch, A. and Geller, G. (1996) 'Feminism, bioethics, and genetics', in S. M. Wolf (ed.), *Feminism and Bioethics: Beyond reproduction*, New York: Oxford University Press.

Bailey, R. (1996) 'Prenatal testing and the prevention of impairment: a woman's right to choose?', in J. Morris (ed.), *Encounters with Strangers: Feminism and disability*, London: Women's Press.

Barker, D. (1989) 'The biology of stupidity: genetics, eugenics and mental deficiency in the interwar years', *British Journal for the History of Science*, 22, pp. 347–75.

Bateson, P. and Martin, P. (1999) *Design for a Life*, London: Jonathan Cape.

Beck-Gernsteim, E. (1990) 'Changing duties of parents: from education to bio-engineering?', *International Social Science Journal*, 42, pp. 451–63.

Berger, A. (1999) 'Private company wins rights to Icelandic gene database', *British Medical Journal*, 318, p. 11.

BMA (1992) *Our Genetic Future: The science and ethics of genetic technology*, Milton Keynes: Open University Press.

Bobrow, M. and Thomas, S. (2001) 'Patents in a genetic age', *Nature*, 407, pp. 763–4.

British Society for Human Genetics (1999) 'Co-ordinated arrangements for genetic testing for rare disorders'. See http://www.bham.ac.uk/BSHG/raredis.htm.

Britton, J. and Knox, A. J. (1991) 'Screening for cystic fibrosis', *Lancet*, 388, p. 1524.

Broberg, G. and Roll-Hansen, N. (eds) (1996) *Eugenics and the Welfare State: Sterilization policy in Denmark, Sweden, Norway and Finland*, East Lansing, MI: Michigan State University Press.

Broberg, G. and Tydén, M. (1996) 'Eugenics in Sweden: efficient care', in G. Broberg and N. Roll-Hansen (eds), *Eugenics and the Welfare State: Sterilization policy in Denmark, Sweden, Norway and Finland*, East Lansing, MI: Michigan State University Press.

Buchanan, A., Brock, D., Daniels, N. and Wikler, D. (2000) *From Chance to Choice: Genetics and justice*, Cambridge: Cambridge University Press.

Burleigh, M. (1994) *Death and Deliverance: 'Euthanasia' in Germany 1900–1945*, Cambridge: Cambridge University Press.

Burleigh, M. (1997) *Ethics and Extermination: Reflections on Nazi genocide*, Cambridge: Cambridge University Press.

Caplan, A. L. (1994) 'Handle with care: race, class and genetics', in T. F. Murphy and M. A. Lappé (eds), *Justice and the Human Genome Project*, Berkeley: University of California Press.

Caplan, A. L., McGee, G. and Magnus, D. (1999) 'What is immoral about eugenics?' *British Medical Journal*, 319, p. 1284.

Chadwick, R. (1999) 'The Icelandic database: do modern times need modern sagas?', *British Medical Journal*, 319, pp. 441–4.

Clarke, A. (1991) 'Is non-directive genetic counselling possible?', *Lancet*, 338, pp. 998–1000.

Clarke, A. (ed.) (1994) *Genetic Counselling: Practice and principles*, London: Routledge.

Clarke, A. and Flinter, F. (1996) 'The genetic testing of children: a clinical perspective', in T. Marteau and M. Richards (eds), *The Troubled Helix: Social and psychological implications of the new genetics*, Cambridge: Cambridge University Press.

Clayton, E. W. (1999) 'What should be the role of public health in newborn screening and prenatal diagnosis?', *American Journal of Preventive Medicine*, 16, 2, pp. 111–15.

Clinical Genetics Society Working Party (1994) *The Genetic Testing of Children* (chair Dr Angus Clarke), Cardiff, March. Can be accessed at http://www.bshg.org.uk/Official%20Docs/testchil.htm.

Concar, D. (2001a) 'The DNA police', *New Scientist*, 5 May, pp. 10–12.

Concar, D. (2001b) 'What's in a fingerprint?', *New Scientist*, no. 2289, 5 May, p. 9.

Condit, C. M. (1999) 'How the public understands genetics: non-deterministic and non-discriminatory interpretations of the "blue-print" metaphor', *Public Understanding of Science*, 8, pp. 169–80.

Conrad, P. (1999) 'Uses of expertise: sources, quotes and voice in the reporting of genetics in the news', *Public Understanding of Science*, 8, pp. 285–302.

Cook-Deegan, R. (1994) *The Gene Wars: Science, politics and the human genome*, New York: W. W. Norton.

Cowan, R. S. (1994) 'Women's role in the history of amniocentesis and chorionic villi sampling', in K. Rothberg and E. Thomson (eds), *Women and*

Prenatal Testing: Facing the challenges of genetic technology, Columbus, OH: Ohio State University Press.

Cranor, C. F. (ed.) (1994) *Are Genes Us? The social consequences of the new genetics*, New Brunswick, NJ: Rutgers University Press.

Cravens, H. (1978) *The Triumph of Revolution: American scientists and the hereditary–evolutionary controversy, 1900–1941*, Philadelphia: University of Pennsylvania Press.

Crow, L. (1996) 'Including all of our lives: renewing the social model of disability', in J. Morris (ed.), *Encounters with Strangers: Feminism and disability*, London: Women's Press.

Curtis, J. R., Burke, W., Kassner, A. W. and Aitken, M.L. (1997) 'Absence of health insurance is associated with decreased life expectancy in patients with cystic fibrosis', *American Journal of Respiratory and Critical Care Medicine*, 155, 6, pp. 1921–4.

Davis, B. D. (ed.) (1992) *The Genetic Revolution: Scientific prospects and human perceptions*, Baltimore, MD: Johns Hopkins Press.

Davis, D. (2001) *Genetic Dilemmas: Reproductive technology, parental choices and children's futures*, New York: Routledge.

Davison, A., Barns, I. and Schibeci, R. (1997) 'Problematic publics: a critical review of surveys of public attitudes to biotechnology', *Science, Technology and Human Values*, 22, 3, pp. 317–48.

Davison, C. (1996) 'Predictive genetics: the cultural implications of supplying probable futures', in T. Marteau and M. Richards (eds), *The Troubled Helix: Social and psychological implications of the new human genetics*, Cambridge: Cambridge University Press.

Dawkins, R. (1976) *The Selfish Gene*, London: Oxford University Press.

Degener, T. (1990) 'Female self-determination between feminist claims and "voluntary" eugenics, between "rights" and ethics', *Journal of International Feminist Analysis*, 3, 2, 87–99.

DeGrandpre, R. (2000) *Ritalin Nation: Rapid-fire culture and the transformation of human consciousness*, New York: Norton.

Dobson, R. (2000) 'Gene therapy saves immune deficient babies in France', *British Medical Journal*, 320, p. 1225.

Drouard, A. (1998) 'On eugenicism in Scandinavia', *Population*, 53, 3, pp. 633–42.

Duster, T. (1990) *Backdoor to Eugenics*, New York: Routledge.

Duster, T. and Beeson, D. (2001) *Pathways and Barriers to Genetic Testing and Screening: Molecular genetics meets the 'high-risk family'*, Final Report, Institute for the Study of Social Change, University of California Berkeley, available at http://www.ornl.gov/TechResources/HumanGenome/publicat/miscpubs/duster.html.

Dworkin, R. (1993) *Life's Dominion*, Oxford: Oxford University Press.

Edelson P. (forthcoming) 'Lessons from the history of genetic screening in the US: policy past, present, and future', in P. Boyle and K. Nolan (eds), *Setting Priorities for Genetic Services*, Washington, DC: Georgetown University Press.

Emery, A. (1968) 'Genetics in medicine', University of Edinburgh Inaugural Lecture, no. 35.

Farrall, L. (1970) 'The origins and growth of the English eugenics movement, 1865–1925', PhD thesis, University of Indiana.

Farrant, W. (1985) 'Who's for amniocentesis?' in H. Homans (ed.), *The Sexual Politics of Reproduction*, London: Gower.

Fraser, S. (ed.) (1995) 'Introduction', *The Bell Curve Wars: Race, intelligence and the future of America*, New York: Basic Books.

Friedlander, H. (1995) *The Origins of Nazi Genocide: From euthanasia to the Final Solution*, Chapel Hill and London: University of North Carolina Press.

Fujimura, J. (1988) 'The molecular bandwagon in cancer research: where social worlds meet', *Social Problems*, 35, pp. 261–83.

Gallagher, H. (1995) *By Trust Betrayed: Patients, physicians and the licence to kill in the Third Reich*, New York: Vandamere Press.

Gieryn, T. F. and Figert, A. E. (1986) 'Scientists protect their cognitive authority: the status degrading ceremony of Sir Cyril Burt', in G. Bohme and N. Stehr (eds), *The Knowledge Society*, Dordrecht: D. Reidel.

Gillis, J. (2000a) 'Celera to offer data on disease', *Washington Post*, 26 September, p. E03.

Gillis, J. (2000b) 'Gene research success spurs profit debate', Washington Post online, 30 December, pp. AO1–7.

Glannon, W. (1998) 'Genes, embryos and future people', *Bioethics*, 12, 3, pp. 187–211.

Glover, J. (1984) *What Sort of People Should There Be?*, Harmondsworth: Penguin.

Glover, J. (1999) 'Eugenics and human rights', in J. Burley (ed.), *The Genetic Revolution and Human Rights*, Oxford: Oxford University Press.

Goodhue, S. (1913) 'Do you choose your children?', *Cosmopolitan*, 55.

Gould, S. J. (1981) *The Mismeasure of Man*, New York: W. W. Norton.

Graham, L. R. (1977) 'Science and values: the eugenic movement in Germany and Russia in the 1920s', *American Historical Review*, 82, pp. 1133–64.

Graham, L. R. (1981) *Eugenics: Weimar Germany and Soviet Russia – between science and values*, New York: Columbia University Press.

Green, J. (1994) 'Serum screening for Down's syndrome: the experience of obstetricians in England and Wales', *British Medical Journal*, 309, pp. 769–72.

Green, J. (1995) 'Obstetricians' views on prenatal diagnosis and termination of pregnancy: 1980 compared with 1993', *British Journal of Obstetrics and Gynaecology*, 102, pp. 228–32.

Green, J. and Statham, H. (1996) 'Psychosocial aspects of prenatal screening and diagnosis', in T. Marteau and M. Richards (eds), *The Troubled Helix: Social and psychological implications of the new human genetics*, Cambridge: Cambridge University Press.

Gudding, G. (1996) 'The phenotype/genotype distinction', *Journal of the History of Ideas*, pp. 525–45.

Hallowell, N. (1999) 'Doing the right thing: genetic risk and responsibility', in P. Conrad and J. Gabe (eds), *Sociological Perspectives on the New Genetics*, Oxford: Blackwell.

Hamer, D. and Copeland, P. (1994) *The Science of Desire: The search for the gay gene and the biology of behavior*, New York: Simon and Schuster.

Handler, P. (ed.) (1970) *Biology and the Future of Man*, New York: Oxford University Press.

Hansen, B. S. (1996) 'Something rotten in the state of Denmark: eugenics and the ascent of the welfare state', in G. Broberg and N. Roll-Hansen (eds), *Eugenics and the Welfare State: Sterilization policy in Denmark, Sweden, Norway and Finland*, East Lansing, MI: Michigan State University Press.

Harper, P. and Clarke, A. (1997) *Genetics, Society and Clinical Practice*, Oxford: BIOS Scientific Publishers.

Harris, J. (1998) *Clones, Genes and Immortality*, Oxford: Oxford University Press.

Hawkins, M. (1997) *Social Darwinism 1860–1945*, Cambridge: Cambridge University Press.

Henderson, L. and Kitzinger, J. (1999) 'The human drama of genetics: "hard" and "soft" media representations of inherited breast cancer', in P. Conrad and J. Gabe (eds), *Sociological Perspectives on the New Genetics*, Oxford: Blackwell.

Herrstein, R. and Murray, C. (1994) *The Bell Curve: Intelligence and class structure in American life*, New York: Free Press.

Hietala, M. (1996) 'From race hygiene to sterilization: the eugenics movement in Finland', in G. Broberg and N. Roll-Hansen (eds), *Eugenics and the Welfare State: Sterilization policy in Denmark, Sweden, Norway and Finland*, East Lansing, MI: Michigan State University Press.

House of Commons Science and Technology Committee (1995) *Human Genetics: The science and its consequences*, London: HMSO.

Howard, T. and Rifkin, J. (1977) *Who Shall Play God?*, New York: Dell.

Hubbard, R. (1997) 'Abortion and disability: who should and who should not inhabit the world?', in L. Davis (ed.), *The Disability Studies Reader*, New York: Routledge.

Hubbard, R. and Wald, E. (1993) *Exploding the Gene Myth: How genetic information is produced and manipulated by scientists, physicians, employers, insurance companies, educators and law enforcers*, Boston: Beacon Press.

Jonsen, A. R. (1998) *The Birth of Bioethics*, New York and Oxford: Oxford University Press.

Kallianes, V. and Rubenfeld, P. (1997) 'Disabled women and reproductive rights', *Disability and Society*, 12, 2, pp. 203–21.

Kaplan, J. M. (2000) *The Limits and Lies of Human Genetic Research: Dangers for social policy*, London: Routledge.

Kavka, G. (1994) 'Upside risks: social consequences of beneficial biotechnology', in C. F. Cranor (eds), *Are Genes Us? The social consequences of the new genetics*, New Brunswick, NJ: Rutgers University Press.

Kaye, H. (1997) *The Social Meaning of Modern Biology: From social Darwinism to sociobiology*, New Brunswick, NJ: Transaction.

Kerr, A. and Cunningham-Burley, S. (2000) 'On ambivalence and risk: reflexive modernity and the new human genetics', *Sociology*, 34, 2, pp. 283–304.

Kerr, A., Cunningham-Burley, S. and Amos, A. (1996) 'The new genetics and health: exploring lay conceptions', paper presented at BSA Medical Sociology Conference.

Kerr, A., Cunningham-Burley, S. and Amos, A. (1997) 'The new genetics: professionals' discursive boundaries', *Sociological Review*, 45, 2, pp. 279–303.

Kerr, A., Cunningham-Burley, S. and Amos, A. (1998a) 'The new human genetics and health: mobilising lay expertise', *Public Understanding of Science*, 7, 1, pp. 41–60.

Kerr, A., Cunningham-Burley, S. and Amos, A. (1998b) 'Drawing the line: an analysis of lay people's discussions about the new human genetics', *Public Understanding of Science*, 7, 2, pp. 113–33.

Kerr, A., Cunningham-Burley, S. and Amos, A. (1998c) 'Eugenics and the new human genetics in Britain: examining contemporary professionals' accounts', *Science, Technology and Human Values*, 23, 2, pp. 175–98.

Kevles, D. J. (1994) 'Eugenics and the Human Genome Project: is the past prologue?', in T. F. Murphy and M. A. Lappé (eds), *Justice and the Human Genome Project*, Los Angeles: University of California Press.

Kevles, D. J. (1995) *In the Name of Eugenics*, Cambridge, MA: Harvard University Press.

Kitcher, P. (1996) *The Lives to Come: The genetic revolution and human possibilities*, New York: Simon and Schuster.

Knoppers, B. M. (1999) 'Who should have access to genetic information?' in J. Burley (ed.), *The Genetic Revolution and Human Rights*, Oxford: Oxford University Press.

Krimsky, S. (1982) *Genetic Alchemy: The social history of the recombinant DNA controversy*, Cambridge, MA: MIT Press.

Lehrman, S. (n.d.) 'DNA and behavior: is fate in our genes?', The DNA Profiles, www.dnaprofiles.org/about/pgm/topic.html.

Lenaghan, J. (1998) *Brave New NHS? The impact of the new genetics on the health service*, London: Institute for Public Policy Research.

Levine, J. and Suzuki, D. (1993) *The Secret of Life: Redesigning the living world*, Boston, MA: W. H. Freeman.

Lewis, A. (1934) 'German eugenics legislation', *Eugenics Review*, 26, 3, pp. 183–91.

Lewontin, R. C. (1991) *The Doctrine of DNA: Biology as ideology*, Harmondsworth: Penguin.

Limoges, C. (1994) 'Errare Humanum Est: do genetic errors have a future?', in C. F. Cranor (ed.), *Are Genes Us? The social consequences of the new genetics*, New Brunswick, NJ: Rutgers University Press.

Lind, M. (1999) 'Brave New Right', in S. Fraser (ed.), *The Bell Curve Wars: Race, intelligence and the future of America*, New York: Basic Books.

Lippman, A. (1992a) 'Prenatal genetic testing and genetic screening: constructing needs and reinforcing inequalities', *American Journal of Law and Medicine*, 17, pp. 15–50.

Lippman, A. (1992b) 'Led (astray) by genetic maps: the cartography of the human genome and health care', *Social Science and Medicine*, 35, 12, pp. 1469–76.

Lippman, A. and Wilfond, B. S. (1992) ' "Twice-told tales": stories about genetic disorders', *American Journal of Human Genetics*, 51, pp. 936–7.

Lloyd, E. (1994) 'Normality and variation: the Human Genome Project and the ideal human type', in C. F. Cranor (ed.), *Are Genes Us? The social consequences of the new genetics*, New Brunswick, NJ: Rutgers University Press.

Lowe, R. A. (1979) 'Eugenicists, doctors, and the quest for national efficiency: an educational crusade, 1900–1939', *History of Education*, 8, 4, pp. 293–306.

Lukes, S. (1974) *Power: A radical view*, London: Macmillan.

Macdonald, V. (1997) 'Abort babies with gay genes says Nobel winner', *Electronic Telegraph*, 632, 16 February.

McGuffin, P., Riley, B. and Plomin, R. (2001) 'Towards behavioural genomics', *Science*, 291, 5507, pp. 1232–49.

MacKenzie, D. (1976) 'Eugenics in Britain', *Social Studies of Science*, 6, pp. 499–532.

MacKenzie, D. (1990) *Inventing Accuracy: A historical sociology of nuclear missile guidance*, Cambridge, MA: MIT Press.

McKusick, V. (1970) 'Human genetics', *Annals of Genetics*, 4, p. 27.

McLaren, A. (1990) *Our Own Master Race: Eugenics in Canada, 1885–1945*, Toronto: McClelland and Stewart.

Maclean, A. (1993) *The Elimination of Morality: Reflections on utilitarianism and bioethics*, London: Routledge.

Maier, H. (1936) 'On practical experiences of sterilization in Switzerland', *Eugenics Review*, 26, 1, pp. 19–25.

Malakoff, D. and Service, R. F. (2001) 'Genomania meets the bottom line', *Science*, 291, 5507, pp. 1193–1203.

Marteau, T. and Anionwu, E. (1996) 'Evaluating carrier testing: objectives and outcomes', in T. Marteau and M. Richards (eds), *The Troubled Helix: Social and psychological implications of the new human genetics*, Cambridge: Cambridge University Press.

Marteau, T. and Croyle, R. (1998) 'Psychological responses to genetic testing', *British Medical Journal*, 316, 7132, pp. 693–8.

Marteau, T. and Drake, H. (1995) 'Attributions for disability: the influence of genetic screening', *Social Science and Medicine*, 40, pp. 1127–32.

Marteau, T. and Richards, M. (eds) (1996) *The Troubled Helix: Social and psychological implications of the new human genetics*, Cambridge: Cambridge University Press.

Marteau, T., Drake, H. and Bobrow, M. (1994) 'Counselling following diagnosis of a fetal abnormality: the differing approaches of obstetricians, clinical geneticists, and genetic nurses', *Journal of Medical Genetics*, 31, pp. 864–7.

Marteau, T. M., Johnston, M., Plenicar, M., Shaw, R. W. and Slack J. (1988) 'Development of a self-administered questionnaire to measure women's knowledge of prenatal screening and diagnostic tests', *Journal of Psychosomatic Research*, 32, pp. 403–8.

Marteau, T. M., Plenicar, M. and Kidd, J. (1993) 'Obstetricians presenting amniocentesis to pregnant women: practice observed', *Journal of Reproductive and Infant Psychology*, 11, 5–82.

Martin, G. and Hoehn, H. (1974) 'Genetics and human disease', *Human Pathology*, 5, 4, pp. 387–405.

Martin, P. (1999) 'Genes as drugs: the social shaping of gene therapy and the reconstruction of genetic disease', in P. Conrad and J. Gabe (eds), *Sociological Perspectives on the New Genetics*, Oxford: Blackwell.

Mazumdar, P. (1992) *Eugenics, Human Genetics and Human Failings: The Eugenics Society, its sources and its critics in Britain*, London: Routledge.

Medical Research Council (2000) Memorandum to House of Lords Select Committee on Science and Technology, 6 November. Available at http://www.parliament.the-stationery-office.co.uk/pa/(d199900/(dselect/(dsctech/115/115we32.htm.

Michie, S. and Marteau, T. M. (1996) 'Genetic counselling: some issues of theory and practice', in T. Marteau and M. Richards (eds), *The Troubled Helix: Social and psychological implications of the new human genetics*, Cambridge: Cambridge University Press.

Michie, S., Bron, F., Bobrow, M. and Marteau, T. M. (1997) 'Nondirectiveness in genetic counselling: an empirical study', *American Journal of Human Genetics*, 60, pp. 40–7.

Miller, G. (2001) *The Mating Mind*, London: Vintage.

Morris, J. (1991) *Pride Against Prejudice*, London: Women's Press.

Mulkay, M. (1997) *The Embryo Research Debate*, Cambridge: Cambridge University Press.

Müller Hill, B. (1987) 'Genetics after Auschwitz', *Holocaust and Genocide Studies*, 2, pp. 3–20.

Murphy, T. F. (1994) 'The genome project and the meaning of difference', in T. F. Murphy and M. A. Lappé (eds), *Justice and the Human Genome Project*, Los Angeles: University of California Press.

Murphy, T. F. and Lappé, M. A. (eds) (1994) *Justice and the Human Genome Project*, Los Angeles: University of California Press.

Murray, C. (2000) 'Genetics of the right', *Prospect*, April, pp. 28–31.

Myrdal, A. (1968) *Nation and Family: The Swedish experiment in democratic family and population policy*, Cambridge, MA: MIT Press.

Nelkin, D. and Andrews, L. (1999) 'DNA identification and surveillance creep', in P. Conrad and J. Gabe (eds), *Sociological Perspectives on the New Genetics*, Oxford: Blackwell.

Nelkin, D. and Lindee, M. S. (1995) *The DNA Mystique: The gene as a cultural icon*, New York: W. H. Freeman.

Novas, C. and Rose, N. (2000) 'Genetic risk and the birth of the somatic individual', *Economy and Society*, 29, 4, pp. 485–513.

Nuffield Council on Bioethics (1993) *Genetic Screening: Ethical issues*, London: Nuffield Council on Bioethics.

Oliver, M. (1990) *The Politics of Disablement*, Basingstoke: Macmillan.

Owen, M. and Cardno, A. (1999) 'Psychiatric genetics: progress, problems and potential', *The Lancet*, 354, Supplement 1, 24 July, pp. 11–14.

Parens, E. and Asch, A. (eds) (2000) *Prenatal Testing and Disability Rights*, Washington, DC: Georgetown University Press.

Paul, D. (1992) 'Eugenic anxieties, social realities and political choices', *Social Research*, 59, 3, pp. 663–83.

Paul, D. (1998a) *Controlling Human Heredity: 1865 to the Present*, New York: Humanity Books.

Paul, D. (1998b) *The Politics of Heredity: Essays on eugenics, biomedicine and the nature–nurture debate*, New York: SUNY.

Peel, R. (1998) *Essays in the History of Eugenics*, London: Galton Institute.

Pernick, M. S. (1997) 'Defining the defective: eugenics, aesthetics, and mass culture in early-twentieth-century America', in D. T. Mitchell and S. L. Snyder (eds), *The Body and Physical Difference: Discourses of disability*, Ann Arbor, MI: University of Michigan Press.

Petersen, A. (1999) 'Counselling the genetically "at risk": peotics and politics of "non-directiveness" ', *Health Risk and Society*, 1, 3, pp. 253–66.

Peterson, A. and Lupton, D. (1996) *The New Public Health: Health and self in the age of risk*, London: Sage.

Pfeiffer, D. (1994) 'Eugenics and disability discrimination', *Disability and Society*, 9, 4, pp. 481–99.

Pinker, S. (1998) *How the Mind Works*, London: Allen Lane.

Pokorski, R. J. (1994) 'Use of genetic information by private insurers', in T. F. Murphy and M. A. Lappé (eds), *Justice and the Human Genome Project*, Los Angeles: University of California Press.

Porter, M. and Macintyre, S. (1984) 'What is, must be best: a research note on conservative or deferential responses to antenatal care provision', *Social Science and Medicine*, 19, 11, 1197–200.

Potts, M. and Fido, R. (1991) *A Fit Person to be Removed: Personal accounts of life in an institution*, Plymouth: Northcote House.

Prichard, D. G. (1963) *Education and the Handicapped 1760–1960*, London: Routledge and Kegan Paul.

Rapp, R. (2000) *Testing Women, Testing the Fetus: The social impact of amniocentesis in America*, New York: Routledge.

Reiss, M. J. and Straughan, R. (1996) *Improving Nature? The science and ethics of genetic engineering*, Cambridge: Cambridge University Press.

Resta, R. G. (1997) 'Eugenics and nondirectiveness in genetic counselling', *Journal of Genetic Counselling*, 6, 2, 255–8, quoted in Petersen, A. (1999) 'Counselling the genetically "at-risk": a critique of "non-directiveness" ', *Health Risk and Society*, 1, 3, pp. 253–66.

Richards, M. P. M. (1998) 'Annotation: genetic research, family life and clinical practice', *Journal of Child Psychology and Psychiatry*, 39, 3, pp. 291–306.

Richardson, K. (2000) *The Making of Intelligence*, London: Phoenix Press.

Ridley, M. (1994) *The Red Queen*, Harmondsworth: Penguin.

Ridley, M. (1996) *The Origins of Virtue*, London: Viking.

Rock, P. J. (1996) 'Eugenics and euthanasia: a cause for concern for disabled people, particularly disabled women', *Disability and Society*, 11, 1, pp. 121–8.

Rogers, L. (1999) 'Having disabled babies will be "sin", says scientist', *Sunday Times*, 4 July.

Rogers, L. (2000) 'Winston patents technique for "designer sperm" ', *Sunday Times*, 12 October.

Roll-Hansen, N. (1989a) 'Eugenic sterilization: a preliminary comparison of the Scandinavian experience to that of Germany', *Genome*, 31, pp. 890–5.

Roll-Hansen, N. (1989b) 'Geneticists and the eugenics movement in Scandinavia', *British Journal for the History of Science*, 22, 335–46.

Rose, G. (1985) 'Sick individuals and sick populations', *International Journal of Epidemiology*, 14, pp. 32–8.

Rose, H. and Rose, S. (eds) (2000) *Alas Poor Darwin*, London: Jonathan Cape.

Rose, N. (2000) 'The biology of culpability: pathological identity and crime control in a biological culture', *Theoretical Criminology*, 4, 1, 5–34.

Rosen, M., Clark, G. and Kivitz, M. (eds) (1996) *The History of Mental Retardation*, Baltimore: University Park Press.

Rosenberg, C. E. (1997) *No Other Gods: On science and American social thought*, Baltimore, MD: Johns Hopkins University Press.

Rothman, B. K. (1988) *The Tentative Pregnancy: Amniocentesis and the sexual politics of motherhood*, London: Pandora.

Rothman, B. K. (1998) *Genetic Maps and Human Imaginations: The limits of science in understanding who we are*, New York: W. W. Norton.

Rothstein, M. (1997) *Genetic Secrets*, New Haven, CT: Yale University Press.

Ryan, A. (1999) 'Eugenics and genetic manipulation', in J. Burley (ed.), *The Genetic Revolution and Human Rights*, Oxford: Oxford University Press.

Sarkar, S. (1998) *Genetics and Reductionism*, Cambridge: Cambridge University Press.

Schneider, W. H. (1990) *Quality and Quantity: The quest for regeneration in twentieth-century France*, Cambridge: Cambridge University Press.

Schneider, W. S. (1995) 'Blood group research between the wars', *Yearbook of Physical Anthropology*, 38, pp. 87–114.

Searle, G. (1976) *Eugenics and Politics in Britain*, Leyden: Noordhoff International.

Searle, G. (1979) 'Eugenics and politics in Britain in the 1930s', *Annals of Science*, 36, 2, pp. 159–69.

Searle, J. (1997) *The Mystery of Consciousness*, London: Granta.

Shakespeare, T. (1995) 'Back to the future? New genetics and disabled people', *Critical Social Policy*, 44, 5, pp. 22–35.

Shakespeare, T. (1999) 'Losing the plot? Medical and activist discourses of contemporary genetics and disability', *Sociology of Health and Illness*, 21, 5, pp. 669–88.

Shakespeare, T. (2000) 'Arguing about disability and genetics', *Interaction*, pp. 11–14.

Shiloh, S. (1996) 'Decision-making in the context of genetic risk', in T. Marteau and M. Richards (eds), *The Troubled Helix: Social and psychological implications of the new human genetics*, Cambridge: Cambridge University Press.

Silver, L. M. (1998) *Remaking Eden: Cloning and beyond in a Brave New World*, London: Weidenfeld & Nicolson.

Sinason, V. (1992) *Mental Handicap and the Human Condition: New approaches from the Tavistock*, London: Free Association Books.

Skuse, D. *et al.* (1997) 'Evidence from Turner's syndrome of an imprinted X-linked locus affecting cognitive function', *Nature*, 387, pp. 705–8.

Smaglik, P. (2000) 'Tissue donors use their influence in deal over gene patent terms', *Nature*, 19 October, 407, p. 821.

Soloway, R. (1997) 'The Galton Lecture: "Marie Stopes, eugenics and the birth control movement" ', in R. Peel (ed.), *Marie Stopes and the English Birth Control Movement*, London: Galton Institute.

Stacey, M. (1996) 'The new genetics: a feminist view', in T. Marteau and M. Richards (eds), *The Troubled Helix: Social and psychological implications of the new human genetics*, Cambridge: Cambridge University Press.

Stockdale, A. (1999) 'Waiting for the cure: mapping the social relations of human gene therapy research', in P. Conrad and J. Gabe (eds), *Sociological Perspectives on the New Genetics*, Oxford: Blackwell.

Stone, E. (1996) 'A law to protect, a law to prevent: contextualising disability legislation in China', *Disability and Society*, 11, 4, pp. 469–84.

Sutton, H. E. (1967) 'Human genetics', *Annals of Genetics*, 1, pp. 1–27.

Suzuki, D. and Knudtson, P. (1989) *Genethics: The ethics of engineering life*, London: Unwin Hyman.

Suzuki, Z. (1975) 'Geneticists and the eugenics movement in Japan', *Japanese Studies in the History of Science*, 14, pp. 157–64.

Taylor, J. S. (1998) 'Images of contradiction: obstetrical ultrasound in American culture', in S. Franklin and H. Raponém (eds), *Reproducing Reproduction: Kinship, power and technological innovation*, Philadelphia: University of Pennsylvania Press.

Thomson, M. (1998) *The Problem of Mental Deficiency: Eugenics, democracy and social policy in Britain, c.1870–1959*, Oxford: Clarendon Press.

Toy, M.-A. (2000) 'Doctors endorse dwarf abortion', *Sydney Morning Herald*, 4 July.

Trombley, S. (1988) *The Right to Reproduce: A history of coercive sterilization*, London: Weidenfeld and Nicolson.

Van Dijck, J. (1995) *Manufacturing Babies and Public Consent: Debating the new reproductive technologies*, Basingstoke: Macmillan.

Van Dijck, J. (1998) *Imagenation: Popular images of genetics*, London: Macmillan.

Vanier, J. (1999) *Becoming Human*, London: Darton, Longman and Todd.

Wailoo, K. (1999) *Drawing Blood*, Baltimore, MD: Johns Hopkins University Press.

Wald, N. J. *et al.* (1992) 'Antenatal maternal screening for Down's syndrome: results of a demonstration project', *British Medical Journal*, 305, pp. 391–4.

Watson, J. D. (1970) *The Double Helix: A personal account of the discovery of the structure of DNA*, London: Penguin.

Watson, J. D. (1997) 'Genes and politics', *Journal of Molecular Medicine*, 75, pp. 624–36.

Watt, D. (1998) 'Lionel Penrose, FRS (1898–1972) and eugenics', *Notes and Records of the Royal Society of London*, 52, 1, pp. 137–51.

Weir, R. T., Lawrence, S. C. and Fales, E. (1994) *Genes and Human Self-knowledge*, Iowa City: University of Iowa Press.

Wertz, D. (1999) 'Eugenics is alive and well: a survey of genetics professionals around the world', *Science in Context*, 11, 3–4, pp. 493–510.

Wertz, D. and Fletcher, J. C. (1989) *Ethics and Human Genetics: A cross-cultural perspective*, New York: Springer-Verlag.

Wexler, N. (1970) 'Genetic "Russian roulette": the experience of being "at risk" for Huntington's disease', in S. Kessler (ed.), *Genetic Counselling: Psychological dimensions*, New York: Academic Press.

Wilkie, T. (1994) *Perilous Knowledge*, London: Faber and Faber.

Wilson, E. O. (1975) *Sociobiology: The new synthesis*, Cambridge, MA: Harvard University Press.

Wilson, E. O. (1978) *On Human Nature*, Cambridge, MA: Harvard University Press.

Wolf, C. R., Smith, G. and Smith, R. L. (2000) 'Pharmacogenetics', *British Medical Journal*, 320, pp. 987–90.

Wright, R. (1996) *The Moral Animal*, London: Abacus.

Wright, S. (1986) 'Recombinant DNA technology and its social transformation, 1972–1982', *OSIRIS*, 2nd Series, 2, pp. 303–60.

Wynne, B. (1995) 'The public understanding of science', in S. Jasanoff, G. Markel, J. Petersen and T. Pinch (eds), *Handbook of Science and Technology Studies*, London: Sage.

Index

ISSUES IN SOCIAL POLICY

The approach of the Issues in Social Policy series is both academically rigorous and accessible to the general reader. The authors are well known and active in their fields.

Nudes, Prudes and Attitudes: Pornography and censorship
Avedon Carol

Shortlisted for the Women in Publishing Pandora Award

Pornography and censorship have carved a divide in the feminist movement and beyond. On one side is an improbable alliance of pro-censorship feminists – most famously Catharine MacKinnon and Andrea Dworkin – and the moral right. On the other are civil libertarians of various shades and anti-censorship feminists.

Nudes, Prudes and Attitudes is the only UK-based single-author account of the pornography debate from a feminist perspective. It argues strongly that the movement for sexual censorship gives enormous and dangerous powers to the state, promotes the very repression that is implicated in causing sexual violence, and derails feminist discussion of sexuality and related vital issues.

Avedon Carol is a feminist, an activist and a member of Feminists Against Censorship. She is co-editor of *Bad Girls and Dirty Pictures: The challenge to reclaim feminism*.

'a stimulating read' *New Humanist*

'a provocative and challenging book' *Gay and Lesbian Humanist*

'an important statement on the modern feminist stand against the horrors of censorship' *Desire*

'sets out clear and reasoned responses to all the arguments commonly trotted out against pornography' *SKIN TWO*

'What impresses me most about the book is the combination of personal experience, contemporary cultural commentary and historical analysis ... If you only read one book about the crippling dispute among feminists over pornography and censorship, make *Nudes, Prudes and Attitudes* that book.' Dr William Thompson, *New Times*

Published 1994
224 pages, illustrated
Paperback   £11.95   ISBN 1 873797 13 3
Hardback   £25.00   ISBN 1 873797 14 1

Drugs: Losing the war
Colin Cripps

Few social welfare problems have become so pressing in recent years as drug abuse. The spread of ecstasy-taking among the young and the arrival of crack as an international threat have all but overwhelmed the efforts of drugs workers and governments to resist them.

Drugs: Losing the war explains the appeal of cocaine, ecstasy, heroin and cannabis in modern society, and describes their effects on both the user and the wider community. It offers an insight into the closed world of young people's drug use and advocates the provision of an integrated drugs service for young people.

This book does not attempt to be a definitive guide to illegal drugs, although it examines the major drugs in some depth. Neither does it seek to be a comprehensive history or social policy review, a practitioner's guide or pharmacology. Instead it seeks to ask the right questions and to explore the interaction between all these elements that makes the drugs issue such a complex, involved and seemingly intractable one.

The book raises the dilemmas we all need to face in our society. It explodes the myths of the 'drugs war' – those held by both the left and the right, the libertarians and the authoritarians – and argues that a new pragmatism is urgently needed which will challenge those who seek 'quick fix' solutions.

Colin Cripps is the Assistant Director of the Newham Drugs Advice Project in London, and has first-hand experience of fighting drug abuse among the young in an inner-city environment.

Published 1997
176 pages, illustrated

Paperback	£10.95	ISBN 1 873797 20 6
Hardback	£25.00	ISBN 1 873797 21 4

Domestic Violence: Action for change
Gill Hague and Ellen Malos

Domestic Violence: Action for change (second edition) is an accessible and comprehensive account of violence against women in the home, written by recognized experts in the field.

First published in 1993, the book has been fully updated to incorporate recent changes in policy and practice. The key strengths of the first edition – its appeal to both professionals and activists and its grounding within the refuge movement – have now been reinforced by a new emphasis on the impact of domestic violence on children and the development of inter-agency work. The second edition will be welcomed by domestic violence activists, statutory and voluntary sector agencies, and students of social work, social policy and gender studies.

Gill Hague and Ellen Malos are researchers in the Domestic Violence Research Group at the University of Bristol and have written widely on domestic violence issues.

'an extremely useful and welcome addition to the literature ... a basic resource for activists and practitioners which provides a comprehensive summary of current perspectives and developments' Nicola Harwin, National Co-ordinator, Women's Aid Federation of England

'likely to be of value to students, researchers, practitioners and academics ... should be widely read and the findings disseminated' *British Journal of Social Work*

'The strength of the book is in the coverage of recent changes ... reflects insights based on a familiarity with the issue of battering' Rebecca Emerson Dobash, *Community Care*

'If you have ever wondered who said what when about woman abuse, this book will provide the source ... well worth having' *Scottish Women's Aid Newsletter*

2nd edition published 1998
224 pages, illustrated
Paperback   £12.95   ISBN 1 873797 23 0
Hardback   £25.00   ISBN 1 873797 24 9

Antibody Politic: AIDS and society
Tamsin Wilton

The global AIDS epidemic that appeared in the 1980s brought with it a social epidemic: the fear, hatred, bigotry, denial and repression with which the peoples of the world have reacted. The way we, as a society, respond to AIDS is an acid test of our values, our humanity and our social policy.

This book discusses the issues raised by AIDS for every member of society. It outlines concisely the history of the epidemic and summarizes the basic medical information on HIV and AIDS. It then considers AIDS in relation to the gay community, to women and to minority ethnic groups, and analyses its policy implications. From an account of community responses to the epidemic, and of the problematic relationship between the state and voluntary sectors, the book moves to a construction of the probable future and recommendations for personal and political action.

Tamsin Wilton lectures in health studies and women's studies at the University of the West of England, Bristol. Her publications include *AIDS: Setting a feminist agenda* and *En/Gendering AIDS*.

'This useful book explains what HIV infection is, how you can get it and how not to. It might also help you to decide what you think should be done about it.' *Guardian*

'an invaluable guide ... a must for students from a variety of disciplines' *AIDSLINK*

'particularly interesting to those who are looking for a feminist perspective on the AIDS epidemic' American Library Association

'a recommended book ... deserves a place in all academic and medical libraries' *AIDS Book Review Journal*

'an accessible yet sophisticated analysis ... an extremely valuable resource' Lesley Doyal, Professor of Health Studies, University of the West of England

---

Published 1992
176 pages, illustrated
Paperback   £9.95   ISBN 1 873797 04 4
Hardback   £25.00   ISBN 1 873797 05 2

For more information on books published by New Clarion Press:
New Clarion Press, 5 Church Row, Gretton, Cheltenham GL54 5HG
tel./fax 01242 620623; www.newclarionpress.co.uk